1996

Working Together

■

Building Integrated Healthcare Organizations through Improved Executive/Physician Collaboration

■

Seth Allcorn

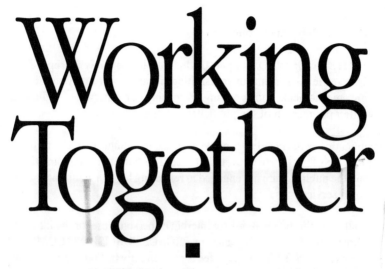

HFMA® HEALTHCARE FINANCIAL MANAGEMENT ASSOCIATION

A **HEALTHCARE 2000** *PUBLICATION*

PROBUS
PUBLISHING
Chicago, Illinois
Cambridge, England

ISBN 1-55738-614-5

Printed in the United States of America

BB

1 2 3 4 5 6 7 8 9 0

TAQ/BJS

TABLE OF CONTENTS

Table of Contents

Table of Contents

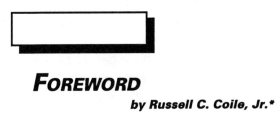

FOREWORD

by Russell C. Coile, Jr.*

On the brink of the reform era, the question for physicians and hospitals is not what Bill and Hillary Clinton are going to do. The real question is what is American medicine going to do to create workable solutions to the nation's healthcare dilemma?

Revolution: The New Healthcare System Takes Shape (1993)

The future of American healthcare may depend upon physician-hospital cooperation. With the collapse of national reform discussions in the Congress in 1994, the momentum for market—based reforms is accelerating. In response, physicians and their hospitals are moving forward to develop local and regional integrated delivery systems and networks. But a legacy of physician independence and mistrust of "big hospitals" could slow progress in the voluntary restructuring of America's health system.

Establishing physician-hospital cooperation won't be easy. Dean Coddington cites two major challenges facing those who would create Integrated Healthcare Systems (Coddington, Moore, and Fischer 1994):

- Are there physicians on the medical staff who are willing to risk their reputations and possible drop in practice in-

*Futurist Russell C. Coile, Jr. is the president of the Health Forecasting Group, of Santa Clarita, California, and the editor of *Health Trends* newsletter. He is the recent author of *Revolution: The New Health Care System Takes Shape* (1993) and *The New Governance: Strategies for the Era of Health Reform* (1994).

come in order to push for the formation of an integrated system?

- Are hospital administrators secure enough in their jobs to dive into the treacherous waters represented by the development of radically new relations with physicians?

If healthcare providers cannot cooperate in developing cost-effective regional health networks, the alternative may be a governmental takeover. With national health expenditures topping $1 trillion and 14 percent of the U.S. Gross Domestic Product (GDP), the voluntary health system is on thin ice. Medical inflation has fallen to 4.6 percent in mid-1994, but will prices rise again, now that prospects for national health reform are fading? American healthcare providers must demonstrate continued competitiveness or they will be hammered by governmental regulation and even a single-payer model, like the Canadian system.

The Imperative for Collaboration

Market forces are driving consolidation, whether the parties are ready or not. Carol Rodat, editor of the Health System Leader, puts the issue of physician-hospital integration directly on the table (Rodat 1994):

"Until recently, many providers were hedging their bets, affiliating loosely with various partners in group practices without walls (GPWW), management service organizations (MSOs), physician/hospital organizations (PHOs), and other cooperative structures. The trend today is moving from looser to tighter arrangements that merge or pool assets so that the financial interests of the partners are aligned."

In the past year, I had an opportunity to make an extended plea in Frontiers of Health Administration for managed cooperation—not competition—in implementing health reform (Coile 1994). There are nine key stakeholders who must be involved in collaboration:

- Physician-hospital cooperation with reforms would reduce potential over-treatment and exploitation of the $50–100 billion of new funding to insure the 37 million uninsured;
- Employer cooperation in enrolling uninsured workers will create stable multi-employer purchasing cooperatives without adverse selection and risk, and create a "level playing field" for all business firms;
- Healthcare worker cooperation through empowerment and "no-boss" organizations would boost productivity, search for practical cost-efficiencies, and enhance customer satisfaction;
- Insurer cooperation in developing a universal electronic claims network would reduce administrative expense;
- Purchaser-provider cooperation under risk-sharing agreements and capitation would further reduce the estimated 15–25 percent administrative burden of the current system;
- Supplier cooperation in mitigating price increases should minimize the need for mandatory price controls;
- Consumer cooperation in compliance and managing a healthier lifestyle could reduce "medical accidents" and preventable health costs;
- Medical education cooperation to produce more primary care physicians and multi-skilled healthcare professionals would meet the increased need for routine care which national access/reforms will create; and
- Government cooperation between the administration, congress, and judicial branches is badly needed to break the "gridlock" funding health access, expanded support for badly-needed public health and wellness programs, reform of the malpractice system, antitrust relief for regional provider networks, and reduced government regulation.

Calls for Cooperation—Not Competition

Seth Allcorn's *Working Together* is a call for a cooperative approach to voluntary regionalization of health services. It will be local—not Washington-based—reform initiatives over the next five to seven years which will move America forward in rationalizing care and making incremental progress on access issues. Allcorn's appeal for cooperation is based on a multistakeholder approach which would establish a durable partnership between the major parties who have a stake in reforming America's $1 trillion dollar health system.

Without being overly dramatic, Seth Allcorn's belief in cooperative implementation of healthcare restructuring could be the last, best hope of a voluntary American system. My Frontiers argument for "managed cooperation" in healthcare is based on the belief that, fundamentally, health is more social service than market commodity. But without the Clinton plan and national legislation for health insurance, the reform initiative shifts to the market. The solution for the excesses of competition, such as surplus capacity and high administrative costs, is to engage in a multi-party structural reform by all major stakeholders—the public, elected officials, insurers and managed care plans, hospitals, physicians and other health professionals, major and small employers, and government.

The Keystone of Physician-Hospital Cooperation

First, we must learn how physicians and their hospitals can work together. Seth Allcorn's *Working Together* is a guidebook to a new era in physician-hospital relations. From his experience in academic medical centers, Allcorn is all too familiar with the stresses which pull doctors and their hospitals in differnet directions. The imperative for integration is very evident from the perspective of the academic center, which is often the organizing force for "hub-and-spoke" regional networks in tomorrow's healthcare delivery systems.

Hospitals are, by their nature, social organizations with a complex culture. Understanding the differences between physician and management perspectives is vital to creating organizational bridges for collaboration. The future of America's hospitals hangs in the balance. Promoting collaboration between physicians and their hospitals is vital to the continuation of this nation's unique community-based system. Chapter 2, "Understanding Healthcare Executives and Physician Executives," is worth the entire price of this book for its insights into the innate psychological differences between these essential partners. Chapter 7, "The Foundation of Network Culture," establishes the cooperative basis for creating tomorrow's horizontally and vertically integrated delivery systems. Chapter 9, "Managing Organizational Culture," is a primer on the development of much-needed regional delivery systems.

Seth Allcorn brings 20 years of experience to the task of strengthening the fragile coalition between U.S. hospitals and their medical staff. Many physicians are still experiencing Kubler Ross' stages of grieving, and are not yet ready for accommodation and cooperation in the restructuring of healthcare delivery. That attitude must change, and quickly, or hospitals and their doctors may miss windows of opportunity. Tomorrow's regional delivery systems are being constructed rapidly now. The hourglass has been tipped, and the sand is running for development of integrated healthcare systems. The time for physician-hospital cooperation is now!

Sources

Coddington, Dean A., Keith D. Moore, and Elizabeth A. Fischer. *Integrated Health Care: Reorganizing the Physician, Hospital, and Health Plan Relationship.* Englewood, CO: Center for Research in Ambulatory Health Care Administration, 1994.

Coile, Russell C., Jr. "Managed Cooperation—Not Competition—to Implement Health Reform," *Frontiers of Health Administration,* 10(3) (Spring 1994): 3–28.

————. *Revolution: The New Health Care System Takes Shape.* Knoxville, TN: Whittle Books/Ground Rounds Press.

Rodat, Carol. "Primary Care Development Strategies," *Health System Leader,* 1 (April 1994): 1–18.

PREFACE

Working together is not always easy and can, in fact, become very difficult when healthcare and physician executives are placed under considerable stress, as is the case these days in the healthcare industry. Hospitals, medical groups, and free-standing healthcare facilities such as laboratories and rehabilitative and long-term care organizations accomplish fine work, but often have difficulty getting employees, departments, programs, and managers to work together to provide high-quality, patient-friendly, and cost-effective services. The same holds true for academic health sciences centers with their complex array of schools of medicine, dentistry, nursing, and allied health, and associated university and affiliated teaching hospitals.

The difficulty of working together within these organizations is still less severe than working with other hospitals, medical groups, and freestanding facilities and services. The ability for many healthcare delivery organizations to cooperate and collaborate will, however, become a necessity in the future as huge regional horizontally and vertically integrated healthcare delivery networks emerge. Cooperation and collaboration will be the foundation upon which these networks will build fully integrated information and service systems that permit the delivery of seamless patient care throughout the network. Another important network-building task that will tax trust and collaboration is the need to rationalize the network's resources by eliminating duplication and excess capacity and adding needed services. These types of major change will test the best of collaborative relationships. These tough networking tasks will demand much give-and-take among managements of the organizations participating in the network and even the development of some altruism. These considerations make it clear that being able to work together effectively is going to be the key in what will become extraordinarily large and complex multibillion dollar businesses.

The problem of working together to produce an outstanding networking outcome is, however, often more difficult than merely developing a plan or detailed set of written instructions. How people feel and what they think often gets in the way of progress. Executives and staff can become unaccountably resistant to making changes and "organization politics" (which have as their goal influencing events and perhaps acquiring sufficient power to control them) may abound. Every hospital and medical group has as part of its history, culture, and mythology horror stories about failures that could have been avoided. A hospital opens a new bone marrow transplant unit one day and then closes it a few days later due to a lack of willingness of several executives to deal with staffing. A medical group invests heavily in one powerful physician's vision only to have the physician leave and take with him colleagues who were recruited at great expense.

Hospitals and medical groups are not alone in these problems. The many parts of academic health sciences centers also have problems in working together. A number of clinical chairs are suddenly fired by a dean who does not like them and who subsequently has to reappoint many of them because the institution has insufficient resources to recruit new chairs. A number of new buildings are planned without considering whether the infrastructure (steam, electrical power, sewers) is available to support them or whether there will be sufficient resources to operate the buildings once they are built.

These unfortunate outcomes and many others gradually led me to look away from management books for answers as to why these problems occur. These horror stories and thousands of others that have or will occur in hospitals and medical groups are very often avoidable if the people who run them are better prepared to work together within their organization and with the leaders of other organizations.

This book is devoted to exploring why healthcare and physician executives often have a hard time working with each other. In particular, this book is devoted to understanding the psychological side of building and operating horizontally and vertically integrated healthcare delivery networks. The psychological side of work is not often covered to much extent in graduate school management courses because it deals with unconsciously motivated behavior and organizational dynamics. This book, however, has as its goal providing healthcare and physician executives psychological insights into themselves and their leadership styles as well as into their colleagues and their leadership styles. Greater awareness and understanding of this most important aspect of the human side of work will make developing fully integrated networks and improving their operation easier for those who have the onerous responsibility of leading the way.

The discussion of the psychological side of work is made accessible in this book by avoiding as much psychological jargon as possible. Even so, it is easy to be skeptical about this approach to understanding organizational life and dynamics. In an effort to overcome some of this skepticism, I want to take a moment to share with you my reasons for believing why the content of this book is important for healthcare and physician executives.

During the past twenty years, I have served as a senior executive in three academic health sciences centers that are, in a way, long-standing examples of efforts to develop horizontally and vertically integrated healthcare delivery organizations. These centers struggle to find ways to successfully combine the elements of a fully integrated network while including other potentially conflicting missions such as teaching and research. These huge, high-tech, tertiary care centers have had to learn to integrate the work of physicians caring for their patients with the cost-effective operation of university hospitals in order to compete in the managed care marketplace. They have also built a network of teaching-affiliated hospitals and, developed networks of satellite clinics and practice sites, and health plans such as PPOs and HMOs. In this regard, they share many of the elements of healthcare systems striving for full integration, such as Kaiser Permanente, Henry Ford in Detroit, UniHealth America in Los Angeles, and the Geisinger System in Pennsylvania to list a few.

Working in academic health sciences centers has been exciting and challenging. Much of the challenge derives from the extraordinary complexity in academic health sciences centers that often calls for balancing the interests of clinical and basic science departments; other schools such as nursing, dentistry, and Allied Health; large teaching hospitals; centralized physician practice plans; ambulatory facilities; other affiliated hospitals and physician practices; the university and state legislature; and accrediting bodies and the federal government, while also offering user-friendly, high-tech, but cost-effective services to patients in a growing competitive and managed care environment. I put all of the above into one sentence to underscore the complex linkage of these elements. Such complexities can lead to slow decision making because many, if not all, of these interdependent elements must be considered and balanced.

This complexity is inherent in the development of fully integrated networks. Developing networks must deal with a vast array of complicated federal and state laws and regulations; financing; contracting; patient, financial, and management information systems; negotiations with potential members of the network, including insurance plans; and the responses of competitors.

The complexity, however, is, in my opinion, often equalled by yet another element: the nature of the people who must create and operate these fully integrated networks. Healthcare executives, while having their share of unconsciously motivated behavior, are nonetheless often better prepared for the new networked operating environment than their physician executive colleagues. Healthcare executives, while encountering problems in working together, are, in final analysis, used to working in a complex and interdependent management milieu. In contrast, physician executives are often not prepared to be executives who must lead and administrate. They seldom receive training and frequently end up patching together management methods and leadership styles they have seen admired mentors and others use, which frequently results in their creating leadership and administrative styles uniquely suited to their personalities. As a result, the most complex organizations on earth are in part developed and operated by individuals who are the least prepared to manage them.

It is this aspect of organizational life, the uniqueness of the personality of each healthcare and physician executive, that casts an extraordinarily long shadow across efforts to work together to develop and manage fully integrated networks. There are inevitably many irrationalities introduced into planning, decision making, implementation, and operations.

Given the nature and complexity of organizational leadership and management, I began to realize that developing sound information systems to support decision making, developing a meaningful list of alternatives for problem solving, selecting a solution, and then monitoring its progress did not necessarily apply in many instances to a healthcare system that was for many years encouraged to be less than well managed by cost reimbursement. I noticed that unnecessary facilities were occasionally built and that facilities were renovated and later had to be changed. The lack of comprehensive long-range planning in many instances led to opportunistic problem solving using the mix of variables available at the moment. I also observed that some healthcare executives and physicians acquired roles that they used to try to dominate and control what was going on because they were anxious about what their colleagues were doing. And it was clear that decisions were often made based on a history of friendship or conflict rather than on the facts.

The solutions to these problems are not to be found in schools of management. As a result, I began a long journey to learn what I could about these types of organizational dynamics.

In the mid 70s, I began reading books about bureaucracy. I gained a much better appreciation of the pervasiveness of dysfunctional organizational behavior. The case studies, research, and stories were at times amusing but also disheartening for someone who wanted to improve matters. Although illuminating, the books did not answer the question of why people act the way they do at work. Eventually, in the early 80s, I discovered that psychoanalytic theory provides a rich theoretical perspective for understanding the psychological, unconscious, and often irrational side of the workplace.

Psychoanalytic theory is actually not one theory, but many theoretical perspectives that shed light on human development and subsequent functioning. Books dealing with this subject matter often use complicated concepts and confusing jargon that can cause the uninformed reader to stop reading. In this book, however, I have tried to present psychoanalytically informed perspectives that are easy to read and understand.

It is also important to appreciate that much of what is covered in this book is a part of learning that takes place on the job. Organization members quickly learn a whole raft of unwritten rules about how the organization works and about many of the idiosyncracies of the executives who operate them. A new employee may be warned not to cross a manager who is known to be a hot head. The employee may quickly learn that, despite being told to take the initiative, all decisions have to be approved by one senior executive or perhaps that no one really makes any decisions at all. Polarized subgroups may exist that do not always work to fulfill the organization's mission, if it is even known. The list could go on. The point is that in one way or another everyone at work has to deal with the psychological side of the workplace and it is better to have an understanding of it than to merely wade into it and try to deal with it on an ad hoc basis.

In sum, healthcare and physician executives are entering an epoch unlike anything thus far encountered. It will be stressful, and many personal and professional beliefs that inhibit the development of fully integrated networks will have to be confronted. This is going to mean a lot of change and accompanying loss, pain, and resistance for everyone. Hospital executives and governing boards will lose autonomy and, in many instances, control of their hospitals. Their hospitals will very likely have to modify and perhaps close some of their programs, all in the name of optimizing the system. Physicians will also lose autonomy and will be asked to change practice styles, practice more preventive medicine, and reduce the use of hospitals and expensive procedures. There is little doubt that the rest of this decade is going to be exceptionally stressful for network, healthcare and physician executives, which will create problems in working together to build, operate, expand, and optimize a fully integrated network.

I hope you will enjoy reading the book. It is the product of my search for better management methods over the years. It is an exploration of the irrational side of work that I have come to believe ultimately dominates much decision making and work when organizational life becomes stressful and people become anxious and psychologically defensive.

ACKNOWLEDGMENTS

I owe a debt of gratitude to my many friends and colleagues in the International Society for the Psychoanalytic Study of Organizations and in particular to Michael Diamond, Josh Rosenthal, Howell Baum, and Howard Stein for always providing me much to think about when it comes to better understanding and appreciating the workplace influences of the unconscious side of human nature. I want to thank Dan Winship for supporting my work and Jean for suffering through my absence from our life together while I developed this manuscript. Last, I must also thank Lt. Savik for her many hours of nonjudgemental companionship while lying on my desk and papers. THANKS TO ALL OF YOU.

INTRODUCTION

Bigger is better in 1994 and beyond. The era of the rugged individual physician or hospital forging out a practice or service area in the face of head-on competition is passing. The ad hoc healthcare system that has evolved, often with the misguided interventions of federal and state governments, has failed to contain costs while providing quality care to everyone. Some crystal ball gazers have predicted that as much as 20 percent of the gross national product (GNP) might eventually be allocated to healthcare if current trends continue. This prediction can be compared to 14 percent of GNP right now, which is already considered too high.

This is not to say that the system is all bad. Despite its costs and access inequalities, it is a system that provides the best healthcare in the world on an episode-by-episode basis. There is no doubt about that. However, there are problems with the system that the Clintons have identified as major issues. The solutions often take the form of controlling costs and social inequity that liberal thinkers believe only the government can ultimately address. Putting aside one's politics, it has to be acknowledged that some of the people some of the time do not receive adequate health insurance coverage or have to become poverty stricken to receive Medicaid to cover costly chronic illnesses of family members.

The issue of access is receiving a lot of media attention. It is clear that the problem is aggravated by loss of employment that translates into loss of health insurance. Popular evening news programs report instances where preexisting conditions are not covered by insurance companies or where limits to coverage are exceeded, eventually leaving families with chronically ill members destitute. Situations like these create moral and ethical questions that are difficult to resolve. Our society is not so wealthy as to be able to afford all the healthcare all the people want. The problems are complex. Americans are saddened, confused, and concerned about the problems they face. These concerns have resulted in a desire for healthcare industry reform.

However, fixing the system also requires funding, which necessitates bringing the cost of the system down so that the savings can pay the additional costs of fixing the inequities. This has led the Clintons and Congress to begin to find ways to alter the system to make it more cost effective.

The movement toward fully integrated regional healthcare delivery networks in the private sector is being encouraged by payer and consumer demands to manage costs and consumption while maintaining access and quality. Throughout the country, the influence of managed care continues to grow. California and the Minneapolis/St. Paul markets are pointing the way to the new marketplace reality. The growth of preferred provider organizations (PPOs) and direct employer contracting have lowered costs. PPOs and some employers have developed enough clout to force healthcare vendors to discount their services in return for the promise of a steady supply of patients. Health maintenance organizations (HMOs), in contrast, rely on a capitated approach. This approach provides a monthly payment to providers in return for meeting all of the healthcare needs of those people enrolled in the plan. This approach creates risks for the healthcare providers who participate because they get paid the same no matter what happens to the health of this group of people. They, therefore, have an incentive to keep the people well; to meet their needs through primary care; and to keep them out of the hospital; which will ironically make its highest profit when empty. This approach contrasts to other managed care approaches where fees for services are discounted but the hospital and physician still make their income by seeing patients.

In sum, HMOs and their providers have a clear interest in suppressing the delivery of healthcare as well as providing it as cheaply as possible. However, these interests are balanced by employer interests in acquiring good-quality, convenient care that meets the needs of their employees and by enrollees who, if necessary, are willing to challenge providers over the services they receive in court.

The impact of these marketplace forces have mandated that providers reconsider how they are organized. Competition has resulted in a proliferation of facilities, technology, and services. Hospitals have competed against each other by acquiring the best diagnostic and treatment methods and developing sophisticated programs such as open heart surgery. At this point, the costly duplication of facilities, technology, and services combined with shorter inpatient lengths of stay (LOS) and greater use of ambulatory medicine and surgery have created perhaps as many as several hundred thousand extra hospital beds (400 500-bed hospitals) as well as an abundance of extraordinarily costly high-tech equipment and facilities.[1] Yet another aspect of the growing cost of the system is the oversupply of physicians who specialize in the treatment of certain types of disease processes (they are paid more for this), their maldistribution geographically (they practice primarily in cities), and their growing competition with each other.

When all of these costly duplications and trends are added up, it becomes clear there is a need to better coordinate the delivery of healthcare services. This translates into finding the right balance of hospital facilities; high-tech equipment; ambulatory facilities; physicians by type of specialization, including gatekeeper generalists; and related services such as hospice, home healthcare, and short- and long-term stay facilities for a given geographic area. Also not to be overlooked are health promotion and wellness, which involve working in communities to change unhealthy lifestyles. This approach will eventually include consideration of services not customarily associated with healthcare delivery, such as social services, public health, and law enforcement. A second equally important system attribute is that patients must be able to move throughout the system of providers and facilities as though they are having the services provided by one organization with one medical record, one billing system, and one locus of patient service advocacy (seamless care).

This discussion of the goals of an integrated network returns us to the notion of developing geographically bounded, horizontally and vertically integrated healthcare delivery networks. Fully integrated healthcare delivery networks will have as their goal nothing short of the dominance of a geographic market where ultimately there may only be one major system engulfing many of the preexisting hospitals, medical groups of physicians, and related facilities such as nursing homes, ambulatory care centers, hospice and home healthcare services, as well as perhaps medical supply companies. Major metropolitan areas will gradually see these regional systems develop and it is not likely that more than one major, all-inclusive system, or at best two, will survive within one geographic market. In rural areas, however, there will be only one. These considerations lead to the need to further explore what is meant by a fully integrated network.

The Meaning of Integration

Developing or participating in regional vertically and horizontally integrated healthcare delivery networks has become the focus of many healthcare providers who are seeking to survive in the evolving marketplace where access, efficiency, effectiveness, low cost, quality, and user-friendliness are the goals. Vertical integration is a concept that when applied to an industry such as steel, translates into acquiring or controlling the mines that produce the raw materials; the means of transporting the raw materials; the plants that process the raw materials into steel; and the sales force to market the steel, possibly including ownership or control of end user companies.

In the healthcare industry, vertical integration translates into a comprehensive system of providers that includes physicians who control the diagnosis and treatment of disease, their offices, and related ambulatory facilities. It includes hospitals, home healthcare organizations, and long-term care facilitates that contain a mixed levels of care for the elderly. Vertical integration will also eventually include wellness, social work, public health programs, and a financing organization such as an HMO.

Vertical integration can be compared to its allied concept, horizontal integration, where a steel mill builds or acquires more and more steel mills or a hospital chain acquires more and more hospitals on a regional or national basis. Networks will acquire multiple hospitals and medical groups in order to strategically place resources geographically to insure easy access. The end product of vertical and horizontal integration efforts in the 1990s is intended to be a fully integrated regional healthcare delivery system that includes all of the resources in the proportion required to meet the healthcare needs of those who live and work within its geographic boundaries.

Developing a fully integrated healthcare delivery network that assembles the right mix of physicians, equipment, and facilities that are evenly distributed throughout the market, however, is no small challenge. Everyone in the marketplace will want to be a player at the bargaining table out of fear that exclusion will mean loss of market share and failure to thrive. This will be particularly important for academic health sciences centers, which must be prepared to become cost-effective, patient-friendly, care providers, constituting the hub of a huge regional system that must cover millions of lives in order to be viable.

The development of integrated networks requires the careful assembly of physicians, facilities, services, and supporting systems. It also requires the reorganization of the system's resources to become more cost-effective. This translates into physicians and hospitals changing what they do in the spirit of optimizing the entire system rather than just their practice or hospital. It means physician medical groups and hospitals have to expand or contract at the direction of the system. Hard-won open heart surgical programs may have to be closed and all such services provided at one or two sites where sufficient volume makes them cost-effective while improving quality.

These networked organizations of the future will look and operate differently. Figure 1 depicts the present healthcare system with its many freestanding, uncoordinated, and highly competitive hospitals, medical groups, long-term care facilities, and other related services. The system looks disorganized because it is. Duplication and excess capacity is encouraged, as is the search for new patients and new illnesses to treat.

Figure 2 depicts the nature of a fully integrated network. The hospitals, medical groups, long-term care facilities, and other ancillary services are carefully organized both in terms of geography and in terms of the services they offer to balance the system and

---

Figure 1   Current Healthcare System

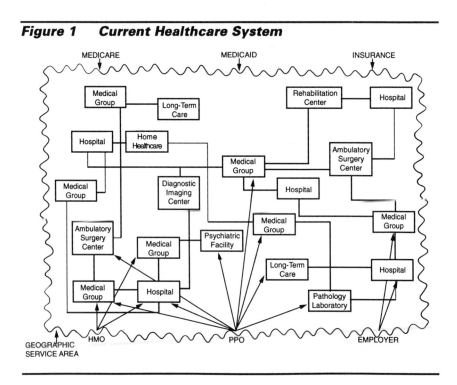

Figure 2   Fully Integrated Regional Network

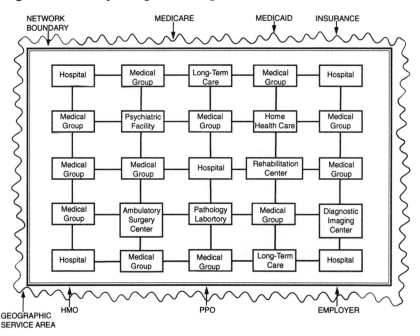

minimize excess capacity and duplication. Accomplishing this is a demanding challenge for the future.

Figure 3 depicts the nature of governance of a fully integrated network. There are many possible ways to go about designing the governance and structure of a network. Figure 3 illustrates the basic elements of integration, which bring together hospitals and physicians with a third organization that represents the network.

Figure 4 depicts a fully integrated network in the form of an organization chart. In this case, a foundation forms the basis for the network, which then owns or controls multiple hospitals, medical groups and practice sites, a health plan, a corporate management system, and service and ancillary service institutions. What is important to appreciate is that negotiations among participants to develop and manage a fully integrated network will be filled with conflicting motivations, making the process extremely challenging and stressful.

Figure 3   *Network Structure*

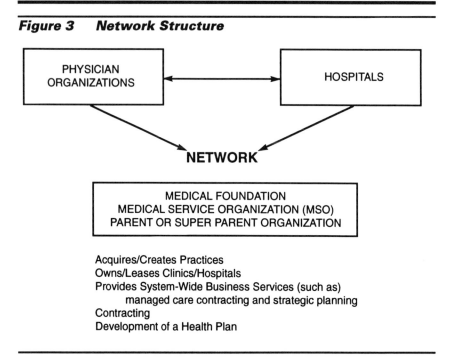

Acquires/Creates Practices
Owns/Leases Clinics/Hospitals
Provides System-Wide Business Services (such as)
        managed care contracting and strategic planning
Contracting
Development of a Health Plan

Figure 4   *Organization Chart of a Fully Integrated Network*

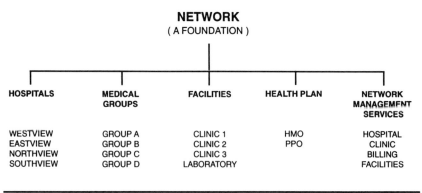

Stress and Anxiety

Stressful situations often bring out some of the less desirable attributes of healthcare and physician executives. When they become anxious, they rely on dependable life-long solutions to cope with their anxiety which often make them less than self-reflective and intentional. They, in effect, become psychologically defensive, and as a result their thinking, feelings, and behavior become more rigid. They begin to rationalize and deny their thoughts, feelings, and actions. As a result, they can become unaccountably resistant, unpredictable, and withdrawn. They may also strike back and become excessively combative and controlling. Appreciating these likelihoods is an important aspect of developing a fully integrated healthcare delivery system. Also to be appreciated is that physicians may cope with their anxiety differently than network or hospital administrators.

This book is devoted to developing a better understanding of the psychological side of working together to create and maintain fully integrated healthcare delivery networks. The success of forming and operating vertically and horizontally integrated healthcare networks hinges on interpersonal relations. The best of logic and analysis can be impaled upon the horns of unresolved interpersonal conflict and distrust.

Physician-hospital administrator relationships often have a long history of conflict. This history is no accident. It is fueled by the different personality tendencies, culture, ethics, values, educational backgrounds, expertise, and management methods of hospital administrators and physicians. The question posed by the movement toward large-scale integration is how this interpersonal and cultural gap can be spanned.

Many examples of the types of problems that must be overcome will be described in this book. However, many of the examples will have unconscious needs for control and autonomy as their underlying problem. Network executives will feel it is important to control hospitals and physicians, who will want to maintain their autonomy. Hospitals will want to try to control physicians who want to maintain their autonomy, and physicians will want to control what is going on to assure their autonomy and income. These often unconsciously motivated trends create a situation where network, hospital, and physician executives may be unprepared to work effectively with each other to develop understanding and collaboration.

Organization of this Book

This book explores the movement toward fully integrated healthcare delivery networks by focusing on the psychological aspects of building working relationships between networks, physicians, hospitals, and employees. Chapter 1 provides a sobering reminder of the many complexities and inhibitors involved in developing sufficient trust and collaboration to build and operate a fully integrated, regional healthcare delivery network. Many of the inhibitors mentioned contain the human elements of thought and feelings, which are influenced by psychologically defensive tendencies arising from anxiety, which is very naturally experienced as a part of the process of integration. In particular, many of the inhibitors discussed in this chapter are understood to be by-products of leadership styles and organizational cultures unique to hospitals and medical groups. These differences in leadership style and culture are critical to understanding the origins of many of the inhibitors to collaboration.

Chapter 2 introduces the psychological level of analysis by providing a model of how healthcare and physician executives respond to stress. The model provides important insights into psychologically defensive responses that are frequently encountered in stressful situations. We all have fantasies, expectations, prior life experience, fears and anxieties, and psychologically defensive distortions to our personalities that affect how we think and feel. When it comes to developing and managing an integrated healthcare delivery organization, these considerations boil down to understanding how we do and do not accept personal responsibility for our thoughts, feelings, and actions. Every executive has been confronted with unexpected, seemingly irrational resistance to planned change. Understanding what makes people who are working under stressful conditions tick is important for achieving success. It is also important to better understanding one's own responses to the distressing experience of anxiety in order to be a more effective leader.

Chapter 3 continues by describing the psychological aspects of the interpersonal world. What goes on in one's mind and how one feels is usually acted out relative to others. This is particularly important for executives who strive to develop interorganizational relations and who are then responsible for maintaining them, which requires constantly solving challenging problems often complicated by unconscious interpersonal dynamics. Effectively relating to others requires developing a better understanding of how unconscious thought and feelings often act to sabotage. This chapter builds upon the model introduced in Chapter 2 and explores the interactions of the different types of psychologically defensive tendencies that naturally arise when stress is present. Being able to work together effectively means being able to understand and respect others, which is facilitated by gaining a better appreciation of what makes people tick.

Chapter 4 continues the exploration of the interpersonal world by focusing on working together effectively in hospitals and medical groups. These important building blocks of integrated healthcare delivery networks have their own unique interpersonal worlds that must also be understood in order to develop an effective network.

Chapter 5 introduces yet another approach to understanding networks, hospitals, and medical groups: group and organizational dynamics. Work, while done individually and interpersonally, is also often accomplished in groups. The new integrated healthcare delivery environment promises to be filled with many groups that will inevitably develop conflicting overt and covert agendas. Understanding the unconscious side of group and organizational dynamics is important for developing an effective integrated healthcare delivery network. Groups and organizations develop tendencies that are difficult to understand and manage. Effectively managing in a group setting will become a critically important skill in the new networked operating environment. A psychoanalytically informed model of group dynamics is provided that explains much of what one finds in groups.

Chapter 6 continues the discussion of groups and organizational dynamics by exploring their nature in hospitals and medical groups. Large, fully integrated healthcare delivery systems will be filled with hard-to-understand hospital and medical group dynamics that can be partially managed by the development of compatible organizational cultures. This chapter focuses the perspectives described in Chapter 5 on these important building blocks of healthcare delivery networks in order to insure that they contribute to optimizing the network.

Chapter 7 continues the discussion of organizational culture and organizational dynamics by focusing on the network as a whole and by introducing the philosophical side of understanding organizational culture and dynamics. Underlying philosophical and basic assumptions about the organization (network, hospital, medical group), human nature, work, the reality of the health delivery organizations, and human relations in the healthcare delivery workplace are described and discussed. Also discussed is how to lead change in organizational culture and dynamics. Successful leaders should posses the key attributes discussed.

Chapter 8 uses the philosophical/cultural concepts introduced in Chapter 7 to understand organizational culture and group dynamics in hospitals and medical groups. Hospitals and medical groups, because they are the building blocks of networks, must be led toward changing their cultural and organizational dynamics to fit the entirely new operating environment created by participation in an integrated healthcare delivery system.

Chapter 9 concludes the book by providing an overview of what network, hospital, and physician executives need to accomplish in order to survive in the managed care, capitated, and possibly partially managed competition environment of the future. Suggestions are provided as to how this work can be better accomplished through psychologically informed organizational consultation in support of change.

In sum, this book provides the reader a lot to think about in terms of what makes large, complex organizations really tick. The reader is provided many insights into how to better manage the many problems and opportunities that exist in developing and operating integrated healthcare delivery networks.

Endnote

1. Surpluses of hospital beds and physicians are seen as one of the major contributors to run away costs. Some of those who have addressed these issues are: Coile, Russell C. "Megatrends 2000: Strategic Implications for Health Care." *Hospital Strategy Report*, 3(3) 2 (July 1990): 1–8; Davies, N. and L. Felder. "Applying the Brakes to the Runaway American Health Care System: A Proposed Agenda." *Jama*, 263 (January 1990): 73–76; Mazique, E. "Trends and Transformation in Health Care." *Journal of the National Medical Association,* 77(5) 77 (May 1985): 365–368.

CHAPTER 1

OBSTACLES TO BUILDING HEALTHCARE DELIVERY NETWORKS

The development and ongoing management of a fully integrated network is a massive undertaking that absorbs the efforts of many healthcare and physician executives and staff.[1] These networks must achieve cost effectiveness in managing the health and well-being of many hundreds of thousands, if not millions, of covered lives distributed across large cities or vast areas of less densely populated regions. Fully integrated networks will encompass a number of hospitals; many medical groups, physicians, and practice sites; long-term care facilities; sophisticated home healthcare services; rehabilitation and educational services; same-day surgery centers; imaging facilities; and clinical laboratories in an amount and distribution that meet the needs of the people of the service area. Advanced networks in the future may also expand to include social service programs and environmental monitoring to fulfill their role of health maintenance and early detection for the communities they serve. This list is not exhaustive. Ambulance services may be owned and operated as well as helicopter services. Fitness centers are yet another possibility as well as networks sponsoring neighborhood, community, and school-based health promotion programs.

Large networks may also develop many of their own supply and service organizations such as laundry facilities, waste disposal, pharmacies, and medical supply companies. The list could go on and is only limited by the talents, imagination, and interests of network executives. A fully functioning and integrated healthcare delivery network will tie together many healthcare providers and suppliers of service in a seamless delivery system that provides cost-effective and quality-assured services.

Such an extraordinarily complex and sophisticated system will encounter many stressful inhibitors to its creation. The governing boards, executives, and employees of the many healthcare delivery organizations must be networked into a tightly managed system that rationalizes the use of resources and provides seamless care. This level of integration will make the governing boards and executives of these organizations anxious about their loss of autonomy and control. They will understand that the network will have to optimize the system's performance, which as they see it may not always optimize their well-being or that of their institution. It is these interorganizational dynamics that will cast the seeds of distress and hard-to-resolve conflict, which will eventually lead to anxiety, which eventually promotes psychological defensiveness, which further contributes to suboptimizing system performance.

The development of fully integrated regional healthcare delivery networks must be understood to be the integration of boards, executives, and employees and not merely organizations and facilities. Every affiliation, merger, or buyout is most importantly a change for the boards, executives, and employees of the hospital, medical group, or other ancillary organization or service being integrated. Change represents loss of control and the introduction of accompanying uncertainty and anxiety. There are many uncertain gains and losses for those undergoing change. Anyone who has lived through their organization being downsized, merged, or bought out knows the many thoughts and feelings provoked by change. Frustration, anxiety, fear, and anger often flood the organization. It is, therefore, understandable that the executives responsible for negotiating the integration of their hospital or medical group are themselves inevitably anxious about the change they are responsible for imposing upon themselves, their colleagues, and their employees. Often, the closer they come to an agreement, the greater their anxiety, the greater their psychological defensiveness, and the greater their unconscious resistance to creating change.

The hospital and medical group executives being integrated are not the only ones who are anxious. Executives of the network are also anxious. They are anxious about making the right decisions and about the financial resources being committed. At a deeper level, there may also exist unacknowledged aggressive feelings and fantasies toward the executives and staff of the hospital or medical group being acquired. These feelings and the aggressive and even violent qualities of taking over another organization and the inevitable pain that is inflicted upon its members as a part of integration also tend to create distressing guilty feelings that must be defended against. Frustration and anger may also be felt by network executives during negotiations when the executives of the targeted hospital or medical group become anxious, defensive, and resistant. Similarly, frustration and anger are often felt when resistance to change arises after integration. All of these experiences and feelings provide a basis for the development of stress and anxiety. In order to cope with these stressful feelings, one often uses unconscious psychological defenses. Network executives must, therefore, also learn to manage their feelings and psychologically defensive tendencies in order to be effective collaborators.

In sum, network building generates stress, anxiety, and psychologically defensive behavior on the part of executives on both sides of the negotiating table and later on both sides of the management table. Certainly, there are many executives who successfully cope with their anxieties and avoid becoming psychologically defensive. At the same time, it has been my experience that the stresses and strains involved in negotiating and implementing change of this magnitude provoke reliance on the psychologically defensive behavior discussed in this book. Psychological defensiveness introduces dysfunctions into the process of working together that make overcoming the inhibitors discussed in this chapter even more problematic.

Hospital-Initiated Network Development

Hospital initiated network development involves deciding upon a networking strategy and selecting a geographic market area. Many decisions are made about which area hospitals to approach; which medical groups to approach; the nature of the affiliations to be developed; how mergers will be designed and financed; whether to develop a healthcare plan such as an HMO; and which types of additional network resources to acquire, affiliate with, or create. This period is stressful and frustrating for hospital executives as they encounter resistance from those with whom it is desirable to network as well as from competitors. The healthcare and physician executives involved in building a network will have to constantly deal with self-doubt and uncertainty about their plans and work. The following interactions contain inhibitors to working together that must be overcome to achieve success.

Inhibitors to Hospital-to-Hospital Collaboration

Hospital-to-hospital collaboration may encounter many inhibitors with roots in the past. Historically, vigorous competition between two hospitals may have created a combative and competitive atmosphere. The competition may have included devious (at least in the minds of competitors) competitive moves on the part of the hospital CEOs involved, which creates suspicion and distrust that must be overcome. Locating common ground may ultimately leave much ground that is difficult or impossible to cover. The appearance of these undiscussable, interorganizational wastelands may ultimately cripple efforts to work together to achieve meaningful levels of integration. An example is the need to close one of two competing open heart programs, which each hospital's CEO is proud of and feels is better than the other's. Hard-to-resolve conflict may arise concerning closing, changing the mission of, or reallocating satellites and other hospital-owned or controlled facilities. Conflict may also occur among the medical staffs as territory and services are recast into a collaborative and system-wide rationalized approach.

These many potential areas for conflict will necessitate persistent care in working through conflict to capture the synergy of collaboration. This process may, however, be adversely impacted by those who are responsible. The CEOs and other senior executives of the two institutions may have created personal animosities that, if not addressed, will continually undermine discussions, conflict resolution, and collaboration. The governing boards of the two hospitals may also find that their members have difficulty working together based on prior adversarial experiences in these roles or within the community.

Inhibitors to Hospital-to-Physician Collaboration

There are many possible inhibitors to developing hospital-to-physician relationships. Hospital executives generally have limited understanding of or appreciation for how medical groups and solo practices are operated. It is not possible, for example, to have the billing department of a hospital take over billing for a medical group. The two processes have little in common. Similarly, there is often minimal appreciation of the operating culture of medical groups; how they are staffed and managed; how decisions are made; and, perhaps most important, how physicians practice medicine and manage their practice. These cultural and knowledge gaps create situations represented by the phrase, "two ships passing in the night." Hospital executives will find physicians who are interested in personal autonomy and control of their practice frustrating to work with. In turn physicians may look with suspicion at these executives with whom they have had unrewarding interactions over the years and who are now approaching them with networking in mind. In the event the hospital is pursuing a management service organization (MSO) strategy, negotiating the purchase of the practice's assets can become contentious and aggravating. The physicians may seek a price for their assets (equipment, building, accounts receivable, and good will) that is unrealistic and may leave no room for negotiating a fair market value. Resolving impasses can entail each side paying for independent appraisals, which are difficult to reconcile. Conflict may also develop over physician incomes and incentives, how they practice medicine (for example how many tests they order) and how many patients they see in an hour, and the retention of existing employees who are unneeded or can be displaced by hospital employees.

Inhibitors to Hospital-to-Managed Care Collaboration

A hospital seeking to develop a network of providers must develop working if not collaborative relationships with managed care and capitated plans. The hospital will be simultaneously confronted with two opposing forms of incentive: discounted fee for service where it still pays to fill beds and capitation where it does not.

Successfully relating to managed care organizations that primarily seek discounts and limits to the delivery of healthcare creates conflicting incentives and the costly and time consuming accompanying morass of preapprovals, authorizations, reviews, requests for information and monitoring, and billing and collection processes unique to each managed care organization. Physician gatekeepers are placed in the role of restricting care and admissions and seeking the lowest-cost providers. These competitive pressures place hospitals and healthcare providers under insidious pressure that at best promotes cooperation. The threat that the plan will surreptitiously pull its enrollees and move them to another provider, thereby creating a precipitous drop in patients and admissions, is the overarching threat promoting cooperation. However, these coercive, competitive/cooperative approaches to managing the pressures are less likely to succeed than a full partnership in collaboration, which is encouraged by the capitated approach.

Survival in a capitated market requires a systematic approach to keeping people well and out of the hospital and healthcare system. All providers mutually benefit from success. An empty hospital makes more money than a full one. Providers are drawn together by a fundamentally different mission than that of managed care organizations which have as their strategy limiting care and acquiring low-cost services. Capitation draws together all of the elements of healthcare delivery rather than pitting them against each other. Fully integrated networks will be successful in both settings; however, large regional networks are the only method of successfully dealing with the incentives of capitation.

Inhibitors to Hospital-to-Other Provider Organization Collaboration

Hospital executives must be able to develop a vast array of additional services to provide comprehensive and seamless care for the network's clients (employers, plans) and patients. Home healthcare, hospice, ambulatory surgery facilities, pathology labs, imaging facilities, clinics, rehabilitation services, various types of therapies, psychiatric and social services, multi-level long-term care facilities, and even retirement living and fitness centers must all be successfully combined into an integrated network. Accomplishing this can be expected to take teams of negotiators countless hours of effort to either buy, build, lease, or affiliate with the needed resources. Hospital executives will be received with some suspicion as to their motives by many of these organizations which will also be intimidated by the hospital's staff, size, and resources. Building or creating these resources will also be difficult. Competitors can be expected to respond, and rifts may develop in long-standing relationships as more attractive offers are put on the table. The executives of these many organizations and their governing boards will become anxious and defensive about relating to the hospital in a networked manner and fearful of losing autonomy. Also not to be overlooked may be long-standing animosities between the hospital's executives and board members and their counterparts in these organizations.

21

In summary, hospital initiated networks face a vast array of problems, many of which will have as a major component resistance to working together. This resistance arises from anxieties over loss of organizational and personal autonomy and control, which will also promote psychologically defensive responses.

Medical-Group-Initiated Network Development

Fully integrated healthcare delivery networks are also being developed by large medical groups. These efforts have the same goals as those driven by hospitals; however, they evolve in different ways and with different ramifications.

Inhibitors to Physician-to-Hospital Collaboration

Physicians will often view hospitals as a source of funding for their networking endeavor, which casts hospitals in the unenviable role of banker. This is largely due to the physicians not accumulating capital as a result of their drawing medical group earnings out as personal income. This is also understood to be the case by hospital administrators. This circumstance creates misconceptions and tensions as hospitals are pressed into a role of providing capital, assuming risk, and in general being indirectly placed into the position of having to approve and take care of many of the financial and business aspects of network development and operation.

Physicians also have difficulty overcoming their feelings about past antagonisms with hospital administrators. Many of these feelings have existed for a long time, and lengthy lists of grievances and interpersonal offenses readily surface during affiliation discussions. This is especially the case when hospital administrators question the proposal, its funding, and the management of the relationship. Physicians may also not prepare their proposal in a manner and with the level of detail that hospital administrators normally expect. The result is that physicians have a difficult time explaining their proposal, defending its nature, and elaborating its details, many of which may not have been thought through and sufficiently analyzed.

Inhibitors to Physician-to-Physician Collaboration

Physicians understand other physicians; however, this does not assure a smooth and easy process of developing collaborative arrangements. Physicians who reside in a community for a long period of time gradually build up information about other physicians, which leads them to approve or disapprove of them and even develop rivalries and bitter relationships. These feelings can be expected to dominate any effort to collaborate and may even rule out developing a working relationship. Medical groups can also develop unique cultures that dramatically conflict with those of other medical groups. This may be particularly true based on specialty. Physicians and medical groups also develop competitive responses to each other as well as considerable differences in earning power by specialty, which can negatively affect efforts to collaborate.

Inhibitors to Physician-to-Managed Care Collaboration

Physician executives often have misconceptions about the management of large systems such as plans and are often suspicious of their executives who speak in a language and use data that is as foreign to physicians as the work of physicians is to the lay public. Past animosities may also exist over rejected payments and losses from risk pools. Also not to be overlooked is the difficult minutia of day-to-day relations with managed care organizations, which drive up office costs and create many frustrations regarding limitations, restrictions, and monitoring of patient care.

Physicians are also poorly prepared to approach managed care organizations, as they will seldom have the time, interest, or expertise to understand the complexity of integrating a plan into their proposed network. They will not understand the language often used; the actuarial data; and many of the laws, rules, and regulations that are part of the daily work life of managed care executives. They may also be astounded at the amount of data that managed care organizations have collected on them and their colleagues, which they may view as invasive and intimidating. Physicians may readily suspect that they will be taken advantage of during the negotiation.

Inhibitors to Physician-to-Other Provider Organization Collaboration

Physicians are seldom familiar with the many administrative and financial aspects of operating a diverse set of different healthcare delivery organizations, although they will be intimately familiar with the available services and their quality. Once again, past history may be a factor if well-remembered conflicts exist. Physicians, in general, lack a business background that permits them to see commonalities among different types of enterprises. They often do not appreciate that a long-term care facility and a clinical laboratory share the need to manage accounts receivable, accounts payable, and inventories. They will also not appreciate that there are many different types of laws, regulations, and credentialling that must be complied with by these types of facilities. This general lack of understanding and appreciation can lead to disagreement over the value of these enterprises, their mission in the network, and how they should be operated.

Physician-driven networking contains many areas where misunderstanding and hard-to-resolve conflict may arise and create anxiety. The dynamic of physicians controlling the process, however, makes network building unique.

The Evolution of the Network Executive Function

The ultimate evolution of network design and development is the creation of an overarching organization with healthcare and physician executives and staff that have as their mission developing and operating a fully integrated network that transcends the interests of any one element including the original sponsoring hospital or medical group. The development of this new layer of management brings with it mixed blessings. It makes the organization in a hierarchical sense taller, and it formally introduces into the network the network's mission, optimizing the network, which may not necessarily optimize each of its many components' preexisting missions. Network executives also become differentiated by their titles, their power, their offices, and their salaries. They must also inevitably act on behalf of the network, to develop and manage the network which leads to enforcing network expectations and standards. These developments are not necessarily welcomed by all the organizations that compose the network. As a result, yet more inhibitors to working together emerge.

Inhibitors to Network-to-Hospitals Collaboration

The development of a network leads to the development of many conflicts over the roles each hospital should play in the network. Hospital A may be reluctant to upgrade its information systems sufficiently to successfully link with the network's system, while its physicians are reluctant to adopt a suitably compatible electronic medical record format. Hospital B by comparison may have a state-of-the-art information system that is technologically difficult to incorporate into the network, and its staff may be resistant to modifying a system that everyone is pleased with. In these cases, both hospitals compromise the ability of the network to link together all of their healthcare delivery sites in a manner where no matter where the patient goes, his or her medical record is available electronically.

As a result, an extraordinary amount of work and change is required to effectively integrate these hospitals into a seamless system of healthcare delivery that has as its goal optimizing the network and patient interests rather than any one hospital's interests. Much will also depend upon the nature of the relationship.

A hospital that is owned by the network will respond differently than one where there is a long-term contractual relationship or where the hospital is loosely affiliated and may switch networks.

Inhibitors to Network-to-Physician Collaboration

The network may become a remote presence to many of the physicians who staff it. Their relationship may be one of being directly or indirectly employed by the network that will very likely have purchased many of their assets as part of the network's managed service organization (MSO). The result is a distressing loss of personal and practice autonomy on the part of the physicians who may act out their resentment in many passive-aggressive ways (avoiding or forgetting to do things).

They may also resent how they were dealt with when the MSO approached them to buy them out. For example, accounts receivable may not have been purchased at all, as may also have been the case for their valued clinic and office building. They may also resent mandated changes in practice methods, including practice site and volume of production. Conflicts such as these are not forgotten by the physicians involved and, as a result, can severely inhibit working together.

Inhibitors to Network-to-Managed Care Collaboration

Networks may end up developing their own managed care product that competes with other managed care organizations. This can be expected to introduce tension into working relationships with other HMOs and PPOs. Yet another aspect of the relationships will involve the size of the network, the percentage of business that any one managed care organization constitutes, the percent the network holds of any one managed care organization's business, the number of networks in a geographic area, and the total number of managed care plans in the geographic area served by the network. These considerations are competition and control based. Inevitably, this type of Darwinian operating environment will introduce many potential inhibitors into short- and long-term relationships. Each plan will be struggling with its foes as well as the plan of the network, and each network and major provider in the geographic marketplace will be pitted against the other to gain and retain the business of the plans. Finding collaborative space in this ever-changing milieu is difficult.

Inhibitors to Network-to-Other Provider Organization Collaboration

Networks will constantly compete with each other to build a comprehensive network that possesses a good geographic dispersion of resources. This will necessitate either building or acquiring the needed resources such as multilevel long-term care facilities; hospice care; and diagnostic, imaging, and therapeutic facilities. Existing facilities will be faced with several suitors that would like to take them over. They will also be faced with the prospect of the network building competing facilities. Merger or affiliation will lead to losses of local autonomy and control, changes in mission and services, and greater attention to cost-effectiveness and the creation of a seamless system of healthcare delivery.

Inhibitors to Inter-Network Collaboration

Networks will also have to cooperate with each other regarding some services and coverage issues. Occasions may develop in which two networks may combine forces to compete against a third or other networks in the same geographic area. They may also find it prudent to share some types of high-tech facilities or to share in their development. Even though there may be logical reasons for collaboration, there may also be many inhibitors such as competitive stances in the marketplace that are difficult to reconcile, legal problems surrounding restriction of trade, and the personalities of the CEOs and senior executives.

Conclusion

This chapter has served as a sobering reminder that developing the needed collaboration can be filled with many legal, operating, philosophical, financial, and personality-driven problems that can be overcome but not without difficulty. Building a comprehensive, full-service, seamlessly horizontally and vertically integrated, regional healthcare delivery network is not an easy matter. The balance of this book examines the human side of collaboration, which is needed to develop integrated healthcare delivery systems.

Endnote

1. Recent books that help to explain the nature of the ongoing and in many instances forthcoming integration of healthcare deliver are: Bette A. Waddington, Ed., *Integration Issues in Physician/Hospital Affiliations* (Englewood, Colorado: Medical Group Management Association, 1993); Dean C. Coddington, Keith D. Moore and Elizabeth A. Fischer, *Reorganizing the Physician, Hospital, and Health Plan Relationship* (Englewood, Colorado: Center for Reasearch in Ambulatory Health Care Administration, 1994); and Dean C. Coddington and Barbara J. Bendrick, *Integrated Health Care: Case Studies* (Englewood, Colorado: Center for Research in Ambulatory Health Care Administration, 1994).

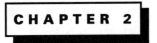

CHAPTER 2

UNDERSTANDING
HEALTHCARE EXECUTIVES
AND PHYSICIAN EXECUTIVES

The psychological side of work is such a pervasive aspect of the workplace that healthcare and physician executives who must deal with it everyday probably do so without realizing it. A colleague is moody, irritable, or withdrawn. During an important meeting, an associate falls into a pattern of blaming others for problems in his or her area of responsibility. The vice president for strategic planning becomes obsessed over minor details that prevent him or her from delivering a report on time. These kinds of counterproductive behaviors, exacerbated by the unique stresses afflicting today's healthcare industry, make up some of the more frustrating aspects of the healthcare workplace. This chapter will help you identify these types of behavioral problems by introducing five personality types commonly found in healthcare organizations that contain dysfunctional elements. Advice is provided for correcting them, particularly when they stand in the way of mandatory workplace changes.

When observing the workplace effectiveness of healthcare and physician executives it is important to remember that, despite their extensive education and training, they, like everyone else, introduce their feelings and personalities into the workplace. All of us, after all, tend to react in certain ways to what happens around us, and our behavior, if inappropriate, can get us off track. Under pressure, we may tend to blow up at bad news, try to control every task we can, look to others for help, or perhaps merely withdraw. Today's healthcare industry, under the gun to change, is indeed a stressful place to work, and it is natural for healthcare and physician executives to feel frustrated, anxious, fearful, and angry.

Because of these particular stresses healthcare and physician executives must develop a keen sensitivity to the psychological side of organizational life. If top-line managers are to be more effective as leaders and collaborators, they must learn to handle the pressures that invariably will affect not only themselves but their colleagues and subordinates. Long-time employees may have to be terminated. They, along with their colleagues, may lose jobs to reorganization. A familiar routine of work may have to change so radically that it might appear that one is learning one's job all over again. How to bring oneself and one's colleagues and staff through these kinds of changes requires appreciating the nature and consequences of psychologically defensive workplace behaviors and learning how to correct those that turn counterproductive.

Overview of the Psychological Side of Human Development

Who we are and why we think and feel the way we do can be understood in terms of nature and nurture. For example, we are all born into the world with certain genetic endowments that ultimately influence our growth and development. But equally important is how we are treated as infants, as adolescents, and as adults. Though it is desirable to receive good parental nurturance and respect, many children are not so fortunate. Typically, these children often respond to the less supportive aspects of their world by developing psychologically defensive responses that help to allay anxiety about themselves and others. These common psychological defenses, such as denial and rationalization (see Appendix 1), which may be employed separately or together, are usually unconscious processes that distort one's thoughts and feelings.

Take, for instance, the case of a child who might believe that by more perfectly meeting parental expectations, he or she will eventually receive their approval, acceptance, and love. This type of powerful, lifelong impulse toward interpersonal control (controlling one's relationship with others) by modifying the self enables the child (and later the adult) to survive and to adapt to an uncertain, sometimes hostile world. But this kind of learned, self-protective behavior, which is facilitated by psychological defenses, comes with some costs. By relying on this type of defensive process, an individual can grow into an adult who, under pressure, has difficultly assuming personal responsibility. The unconscious pursuit of security and the minimization of anxiety may become more important than rationally dealing with an anxiety-filled reality and assuming personal responsibility.

However, the assumption of personal responsibility is, for the builders, leaders, and managers of integrated healthcare delivery systems, a prerequisite for success. It ensures, for example, that healthcare and physician executives—and by extension, their organizations—will detect errors and will develop and change. Unfortunately though, senior level executives sometimes respond to stressful situations by resorting to familiar patterns of behavior developed over a lifetime—in particular, those that minimize their anxiety.

Recognizing these kinds of problems is somewhat simple if you know what to look for. For example, you might find management overemphasizing organizational design and hierarchical authority, which can result in employee disempowerment and losses of organizational vitality. When healthcare and physician executives seek to distance themselves from the negative consequences of their actions (replacing one manager with another, for example), scapegoating the person to be terminated (it is really his or her fault), as a way to defend against anxiety, may become an unconscious defensive tactic. Understanding these complex psychological aspects of healthcare pressures will improve collaboration among executives and management groups and prevent counterproductive behaviors from occurring.

The Model of Psychological Defensiveness

The need to protect oneself against anxiety depends on whether one's professional and organizational relationships promote adequate levels of self-esteem and psychological integrity. If they don't, network, hospital, or medical group executives may feel anxious and, as a result, their ability to assume personal responsibility is compromised, to some extent, by the emergence of psychological defensiveness. When this occurs, their attempts to control their own anxiety often lead to trying to control people and events. These acts of control usually emphasize conformity over spontaneity, routine over innovation, work over play, and disengeniousness over sincerity.[1] At the same time, an executive's ability to assume personal responsibility is lost in the midst of his or her impulse to feel better about him or her self. (See Figure 5, The Model of Psychological Defensiveness)

Assuming personal responsibility implies intentionality. Intentionality involves relatively conflict-free performance where excessive anxiety is not experienced, where grounding in objective reality is sustained, and where critical thinking and self-reflection exist. In sum, intentionality calls for being aware of one's motivations and expectations. However, whenever organizational dynamics turn stressful, one's ability to maintain intentionality and assume personal responsibility is weakened. Stress is typically experienced as an uncontrollable and unpredictable event, which, for example, could occur on the job in the form of an order to downsize hospital staff. The order to downsize creates a sense of loss of control for virtually everyone in the organization and results in anxiety for all hospital employees, including management.

Figure 5 distinguishes between normal and neurotic. Normal anxiety is a reaction proportionate to the threat. For example, it's

Figure 5 Model of Psychological Defensiveness

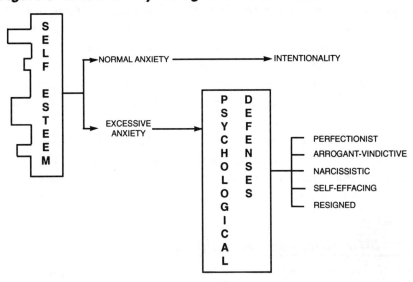

Adapted from: Michael A. Diamond and Seth Allcorn, "Psychological Barriers to Personal Responsibility," Organizational Dynamics (Spring 1984: 66–77).

not unusual to feel somewhat anxious after learning you and your colleagues (as well as others) may lose your jobs during the downsizing period. However, by acknowledging and accepting the news and loss of control and certainty, heavy reliance on psychological defenses to defend against the distressing news is avoided. In fact, those who are not feeling unduly threatened by the order to downsize may interpret the event as a challenge for them to manage.

In contrast, excessive anxiety, that which becomes neurotic, manifests itself as a disproportionate reaction to a threat. This occurs when someone experiences the threat subjectively instead of objectively; that is, he or she personalizes the threat. One's sense of interpersonal and situational control, security, and self-worth are threatened. To return to the downsizing example, if, upon hearing the order to downsize, someone reacts by interpreting the event as a move that will result in the elimination of his or her job, the resulting anxiety might lead to thinking and acting defensively. The employee might react by unconsciously obsessing over minor details or demanding excessive documentation from subordinates before making even small decisions to avoid making any mistakes that might further encourage termination. When this kind of excessive anxiety emerges in the workplace, it can result in either the intentional leadership style or one of five psychologically defensive leadership styles: perfectionistic, arrogant-vindictive, narcissistic, (the appeals to mastery) self-effacing (the appeal to love), and resigned (the appeal to freedom).[2] One of these defensive leadership styles will usually predominate but the others may also be relied upon in an effort to control anxiety.

The Intentional Leadership Style

The intentional leadership style is the ideal executives should strive for. The intentional healthcare and physician-executive is not overly threatened by stressful situations and therefore does not become psychologically defensive. He or she is able to think clearly and is able to observe with reasonable objectivity what is going on. Typical characteristics of intentionality are: nondefensive acceptance of feedback, clear thinking, maintenance of self-reflective skills, sensitivity to what others are thinking and feeling, and willingness to take risks and innovate in the presence of stress. The maintenance of intentionality results in the intentional leadership style.

Fully integrated healthcare delivery networks need this type of leader. The balance of the 1990s promises to be a stressful time for medicine. Healthcare and physician executives who function intentionally under stress will be at a premium. Intentionality translates into being able to make thoughtful and deliberate decisions, a characteristic which is mostly missing in the psychological defensive leadership styles.

The Appeal to Mastery

The appeal to mastery, despite its adaptiveness to many situations is, nonetheless, a psychologically defensive leadership style that has as its aim removing the experience of anxiety. The healthcare or physician executive believes that, by pouring his or her highly mobilized and nearly boundless energy into gaining control of the situation, anything can be accomplished and mastery can be gained or restored. This response, it must be noted, is very likely a reaction to having felt helpless and powerless as a child. Feelings of weakness, helplessness, and dependency are detested by the executive. The appeal leads to three types of distinctive leadership styles: perfectionist, arrogant-vindictive, and narcissistic. One of these styles will predominate; however, the others will also occur depending upon the mix of variables at the moment and the success of the initial style in controlling anxiety.

The Perfectionist Leadership Style

The perfectionistic leadership style results in the healthcare or physician executive establishing what he or she believes is a set of performance standards for self and others that, if met, will maintain or restore mastery. In particular, if the executive holds and perhaps meets the standards, he or she feels superior, which at least in part bolsters threatened self-esteem and provides some sense of self-control relative to the stressful situation. Perfectionists have identifiable leadership characteristics. They pay close attention to detail. They are obsessed with order, rules, punctuality, and appearances. They possess rigid and demanding moral and ethical standards that they expect others to meet.

An example is the attempt to perfect an analysis to replace worn-out ICU monitors. Staff may be asked to test and retest competing brands of equipment and develop numerous purchase and installation scenarios that wring out the last $5,000 of saving from a $4,000,000 purchase. The savings of the last $5,000, however, creates months of delay and ends up costing $50,000 in staff time. The perfectionist often does not know when to quit analyzing and make a decision.

Medical groups also abound with examples of excessive pursuits of perfection. Putting aside its obvious and desirable implications for the practice of medicine, physicians are often critical of others and many business and office practices. Physicians can become preoccupied with trying to gain ever more perfect control of the operations of their medical group and its expenses by demanding tighter control of employees and detailed management reports that encourage them to try to micromanage all aspects of the group's operations.

The Case of Perfect Performance Dr. Jones has a large practice within her medical group which keeps her very busy. She is also responsible for supervising the physical therapy department, which she has little time to do. Her lack of time, however, did not adversely affect the department, as it had a good manager. The manager, however, unexpectedly quit, and her departure plunged the department into chaos. Patients were misscheduled. The quality of service diminished and attendance became increasingly unpredictable for several therapists. Patients began to complain, and a number asked to be referred elsewhere.

The department's growing problems were discussed at a department head meeting and Dr. Jones was embarrassed. Her response was that she would take care of the problems immediately. She met with the therapists and staff as a group to hammer home the point that outstanding quality and service were expected. Having made her expectations known, she went on to say that she would be taking more interest in the department until a new manager was recruited.

She began to drop in unexpectedly to observe the therapists at work and to speak to their patients. The smallest patient complaint or minor deviation in procedure or technique led to a discussion of the problem with the therapist involved. As weeks passed, Dr. Jones's campaign for perfection snared every therapist a number of times. Written procedures were developed or revised by Dr. Jones to guide every aspect of work. Despite improved performance, departmental morale began a free fall. No one appreciated having their work constantly scrutinized. Nonetheless Dr. Jones continued her campaign.

Eventually, a number of therapists began looking for new employment, which Dr. Jones was aware of but did nothing about. She had been heard to say that those who couldn't take it should probably leave. Fortunately, a new manager was hired, and no one left. Dr. Jones thankfully retreated back to her practice. She did not like all of the tension that had developed, and she continued to blame the staff for all the problems.

Intervention Strategy The tendency to respond to criticism with renewed efforts to be more perfect is natural. We all learn that if we try hard enough, we can succeed. The perfectionist, however, takes this pursuit further because criticism is not felt to be criticism of one's performance but rather of oneself. Salvaging oneself takes on emotion-ladened overtones that demand perfection be achieved to save oneself. The outcome is that the pursuit of perfection becomes overdetermined. The pursuit enhances the perception of oneself; while finding fault with others casts them in an inferior light. The perfectionist can easily become the autocratic micromanager who ends up making others feel unable to think for themselves. Those who do not like this atmosphere often transfer out or leave, further reinforcing this tendency (those who are left accept it), which becomes a deeply embedded and undiscussable aspect of culture for the group reporting to this executive.

The leadership problem posed by perfection is to find ways to build upon its positive aspects while avoiding its compulsive use as a psychological defense. This translates into being able to spot its use as a defense against anxiety. When an executive becomes anxious and overly perfectionist and rigid, it is time to encourage him or her to step back from what is going on and examine his or her feelings. In particular, when operating or patient care problems arise, healthcare and physician executives may become overly anxious because they see the problems as a personal threat or criticism rather than as an opportunity for improvement. They may seek to locate who to blame for the problems and greet negative feedback defensively. The result is that the executive, perhaps supported by perfectionistic colleagues, strives for mastery by imposing perfection as a solution to the problems rather than as an expectation for the performance of work.

Understanding the nature of perfectionism leads to designing intervention strategies that avoid losses of self-esteem or attempt to restore self-esteem if it is lost. This translates into making sure that when criticism is offered, it is cast in a manner that is not threatening or embarrassing to the executive. Perfectionism can also be addressed through coaching and training if the pursuit of perfection becomes excessive and undermines working with others. Superiors can intervene by setting firm decision-making time boundaries and discouraging excessive or obsessive analysis. Subordinates can also contribute if they are willing to assume some risk in order to question the constant pursuit of more information and the completion of an ever more perfect analysis. Collective resistance in the form of pointing out that little is being gained by the expenditure of additional energy can eventually discourage the perfectionist from pushing his or her control agenda too far.

The Arrogant-Vindictive Leadership Style

The arrogant-vindictive leadership style results in the healthcare or physician executive seeking vindictive triumph over others who have offended his or her excessive but delicate sense of pride. Personal weakness is not to be tolerated. Competitiveness, winning, and getting even are highly valued. Anyone who crosses this executive understands that a competitive combative response will follow, which may include an avenging rage limited only by consideration of the leader's self-preservation.

The arrogant-vindictive healthcare or physician executive possesses a number of distinguishing characteristics. This leader is dominating, exploitive, and willing to attack and humiliate others. He or she is engrossed in an unrelenting quest for power, authority, and control to bolster self-esteem and protect his or her false pride. His or her style might be described as management by intimidation.

This executive's behavior is easily spotted. A typical example is a hospital executive who, after conducting personal research, believes that he or she has the right and, more importantly, the only answer to a problem. He or she then proceeds to aggressively sell the idea to everyone and, if necessary, is prepared to try to ram the point of view at everyone while also being more than willing to discredit other points of view by any means available. Anyone who disagrees with this executive faces being talked or yelled down and subjected to an ongoing process of humiliation and personalized attacks. Outrageous examples such as these are not uncommon. These executives often have the power to enforce their will; that is why they seek it.

Network, hospital, and medical groups can expect to have some leaders who have a hard time controlling their anger when they are confronted with situations that damage their pride. However, an executive's compulsive mastery-oriented behavior, when challenged or threatened, can be beneficial given the right circumstances. It is tempting to place the executive in situations where his or her arrogant pride and vindictiveness offers a ready solution to problems. For example, an executive's defensive tendency works to a network's, hospital's, or medical group's advantage when he or she is incorporated into a tough bargaining situation. His or her energy and bullying may wear down the opposition. However, regardless of how tempting it is to use a person's defensive tendencies to best advantage, it is better to help the person deal with his or her compulsive behavior.

The Case of Overpowering Leadership Dr. Smith was hired to develop a new home healthcare program. He had years of experience developing similar programs in other parts of the country. He fully expected to achieve rapid success with this new opportunity, and he set about his work with great energy. It was not long, however, before the going got tough. Dr. Smith experienced every inhibitor as a personal affront. His response was to bear down harder on those in his way and to occasionally intimidate them by threatening to get them fired. However, despite the turmoil, Dr. Smith succeeded in developing an outstanding program within budget and on time. The enemies he had made acknowledged that he had accomplished what the network had asked him to do.

Regrettably, Dr. Smith proved to be just as difficult to work with regarding the program's day-to-day operation. He wanted to make all of the decisions and was willing to intervene any time, any place, and with anyone whom he felt was usurping his authority. As time passed, he grew progressively more combative, and it was clear that he was reaching an impasse with many of the program's employees.

He was eventually asked to step down from his role as program director after a major sexual harassment incident with several female employees. This change, however, was publicly presented as a new opportunity for Dr. Smith to develop yet another program. He agreed to lead the development of a new clinic facility from the ground up as part of a face-saving negotiation.

Intervention Strategy The tendency to confront problems and threats to one's self-esteem with antagonistic and combative responses is as natural as responding with perfection. Everyone has fought back against the criticism and actions of others. This response is adaptive up to a point. This point is, however, crossed by the arrogant-vindictive healthcare or physician executive. Problems and threats are found everywhere, which necessitates being constantly on the offensive. Behavior is overdetermined and contains compulsive and unconscious elements that make this executive's response to problems predictably threatening to those who challenge his or her thinking.

The belief that a powerful hospital executive may become vindictive and attack others (yell in meetings, insult others, throw things, and threaten promotions and jobs) is often enough to discourage even the most idealistic and brave of employees from providing nonconfirming information, confronting the behavior, or questioning decisions out of fear of injuring the executive's excessive but fragile pride. This may hold as well for superiors who are not immune to personal attacks and politics aimed at removing them.

Physician executives who rely on this defensive tendency often think nothing of it and may only seem to feel uncomfortable about their actions if they are exceptionally excessive. Otherwise, it is just the way they are and is expected to be accepted. Healthcare and physician executives who must work with a physician executive who frequently develops win-lose interactions will find it challenging. It is important to try to make the physician executive feel comfortable with the interpersonal and group process in order to avoid feeling losses of control, threat, and anxiety. Occasional outbursts are probably best ignored, and an effort should be made to take no offense in order to remain effective at working with this executive. Outrageous behavior, however, should be addressed. In this regard, not doing so may actually encourage the physician executive to rely on the behavior to get his or her way. Care must also be taken to spot the emergence of win-lose dynamics. When this occurs, attention must be paid to drawing the executive back into a collaborative win-win mode of interaction.

Minimizing vindictive responses also involves avoiding threatening his or her self-esteem. This translates into casting criticism in as nonthreatening a manner as possible. Rather than say, "I spotted a mistake in your work yesterday" (implying "You stupid fool"), a less threatening and embarrassing approach might be to ask the executive to double check his or her work because something doesn't look right. However, even in the best of circumstances this healthcare or physician executive will become mobilized and willing to risk a great deal to get even with an offender. When this occurs, coaching the executive toward a less aggressive and offensive reaction can be effective so long as it is not perceived to imply criticism. For example, an executive who is clearly angry about a decision a colleague made might be encouraged by a superior or friend to approach the situation with care and calm to best make his or her complaint known.

Superiors must also make it clear that vindictive and outrageous behavior that bullies, intimidates, and humiliates others is unacceptable. Subordinates are in a much greater double bind; it is difficult for them to have their voices heard, as their superior is always ready to talk or yell them down and consider them disloyal and not team players. Uniform group pressure and interpersonal support can limit the personal attacks and help group members who are attacked. Regrettably, if the executive is highly insensitive to his or her effect on others, the only mechanisms left to subordinates may be appeals to the personnel department, an ombudsman, or to executives higher up in the hospital including the CEO.

The Narcissistic Leadership Style

The narcissistic leadership style results in the healthcare or physician executive striving to appear likeable, competent, and worthy of respect and admiration. This executive is preoccupied with surrounding him- or herself with others who are dutiful, appreciative, respectful, and loyal. This executive is a smooth operator and relies on good communication and self-presentation skills to impress others. This is, in part, achieved by an ongoing effort to essentially purchase these responses through, if necessary, the inappropriate use of organizational resources as rewards. Those who do not respond are punished and if necessary removed. This executive also makes it clear that he or she holds a magnificent vision for the network, hospital, or medical group and generates many ideas in support of the vision.

However, after explaining the vision, he or she prefers to let others worry about implementation.

An example is a male hospital executive who meets with two female subordinates and concludes the meeting by commenting on their attractive clothes and adding that he must be paying them too much. This same executive may promise resources to others such as open positions to fill that are just simply not available in order to appear powerful, important, and worthy of admiration.

Hospital and medical groups are often blessed with so many members with good ideas that they often don't have the time to implement them. There are many examples of hospital and physician executives making plans implementing them without paying sufficient attention to the many problems and details associated with the plans and their implementation. Expensive equipment may be purchased without consideration as to where it will be located; whether the space has adequate power, shielding, water, or climate control capacity; whether there is adequate demand for its use; licensure; the cost of supplies; and the cost of technicians and maintenance agreements. One is equally likely to find major renovations and even new buildings developed without adequate consideration of funding, operation, and staffing.

The Center of Attention Case Ms. White was very pleased to become the administrative executive in charge of the Plainville Clinic. Her predecessor, Mr. Black, had, over many years, built the clinic into a much applauded community resource. Ms. White looked forward to being welcomed into Plainville, and she privately hoped that she could assume some of the highly visible community roles to which Mr. Black had been recruited. However, within weeks it was clear that the clinic's employees and many in the community were not welcoming her as she had hoped.

She responded to what she felt was a cool reception by meeting with many of her employees one-on-one to win them over. She promised her employees new support in their work.

These pledges were well received but proved to be costly, eventually threatening the financial viability of the clinic. She also began to use clinic resources to entertain Plainville village counsel members, the mayor, and a number of influential businesspeople. She was intent upon receiving the respect, attention, and admiration that she perceived Mr. Black had received after 20 years at the clinic. She was not going to be content until she acquired it.

Intervention Strategy Networks, hospitals, or medical groups can have executives with compelling needs to be become powerful in order to feel liked and admired. These are all-too-human tendencies. However, when being powerful, admired, and liked become a compulsive interpersonal agenda that leads to bending the rules and allocating resources, it is time to call a halt to the process. The healthcare or physician executive who tries to prop up his or her shaky self-esteem with external approval is ultimately pursuing a self-defeating strategy of trying to control what others think, feel, and do relative to him or her in order to feel good about him- or herself. When this occurs, being liked and admired becomes more important than getting work done. Failure to gain control floods the executive with feelings of powerlessness and worthlessness. Diminishing these negative feelings is all important.

Minimizing the narcissistic response requires others to constantly reassure the executive while avoiding being manipulated into taking care of his or her fragile ego. Entrapment is avoided by most importantly recognizing that social cues are present, such as the appearance of hurt feelings or some type of injury. Responding may be acceptable if one has an appreciation for necessary limits on caretaking behavior (which implies giving of oneself on behalf of the other). Feelings of guilt must be overcome in the process of withdrawing the support as well as accepting eventual rejection. The inappropriate use of network, hospital, or medical group resources should be challenged when manipulation is evident. It must be appreciated that this executive's pursuit of admiration is foremost in his or her unconscious agenda, even though his or her dysfunctional behavior is contained by watchful supervision and insightful interactions.

Superiors have to constantly monitor this executive's decisions to limit his or her pursuit of power and admiration. Rejection of his or her many promises of resources and support, however, can introduce tension into that working relationship. Rejection permits the narcissistic executive to depict top management as the problem and him- or herself as the good guy who wants to support every request. Subordinates must learn to appreciate that this executive is much more interested in looking good than operating the hospital cost-effectively. Requests made to this executive should be carefully documented in order to survive upper management scrutiny.

The generation of many ideas should not be discouraged. However, they must be balanced by reasonable analysis and attention to detail when being implemented. This can often be accomplished by hiring consultants or adding support staff. In particular, physicians respect the professional development of information by staff experts and consultants so long as it proceeds at a reasonable pace and can be observed to be of good quality. Network and hospital executives must be prepared to provide these services and talent in support of collaboration with physician executives who have lots of ideas.

In sum, dealing with a healthcare or physician executive's narcissistic tendencies requires understanding their origin in low self-esteem and unconscious fear that he or she is not really worthy of admiration or being liked. Self-esteem is easily threatened by the perception of disapproval and rejection by peers and colleagues. Self-esteem is also threatened by changes in job assignments that require recruiting a new support group, as was the case for Ms. White.

Essentially, each of these three leadership styles is a way of seeking mastery over others and the situation to control excessive anxiety and low self-esteem. Lack of control plagues healthcare or physician executives with feelings of powerlessness and worthlessness. Those who recognize and respond wisely to these psychologically defensive leadership styles will help the organization.

The Appeal to Love

The use of the word *love* in the rational workplace may seem a paradox. However, everyone silently hopes to be nurtured and to have unconsciously felt security and self-esteem needs magically met. Leaders who appeal to love do not believe they are capable of mastery and, in fact, abhor dominating and controlling behavior (which they may have frequently experienced relative to their parents). They prefer to let others take charge and run the show, hoping that they will be taken care of in return for their caring, devoted support and loyalty.

The Self-Effacing Leadership Style

The appeal to love results in the self-effacing leadership style. This psychologically defensive leadership style may seem to be inconsistent with assuming a role of leadership; however, a person who puts the well-being of others first, and creates a warm, fuzzy workplace where there is promise that everyone's needs will be met it is often felt to be highly desirable by employees. This response is often especially welcomed when a mastery-oriented leader is replaced. Employees may feel they have been the subject of aggression and manipulation and may react to the opportunity for change by locating a new executive who will be gentle and kind.

This healthcare or physician executive has recognizable characteristics. He or she avoids taking charge and acting assertive when it is appropriate. He or she also avoids dealing with disciplinary issues and conflict. The executive gives few orders and assigns little work, and rarely takes actions he or she fears will threaten, anger, or alienate others. This executive stresses organizational attributes that focus on unselfishness, goodness, generosity, humility, acceptance of personal vulnerability, and sympathy in the hope followers will love and take care of him or her.

The caretaking nature of hospital and medical group work encourages self-effacing leadership. Patients and employees want to feel good and be taken care of. Employees may be willing to accept less mastery of work in order to feel nurtured. Yet, the presence of a self-effacing executive may signal an entrenched group dynamic that makes change difficult. The executive will be discouraged from change not only because of his or her compulsive choice of a defensive leadership style but also because group members do not want change.

Self-effacing leadership may arise anywhere in an organization. A healthcare or physician executive responsible for the expansion of a remote practice site may recruit other physicians and staff who identify with a warm and caring work setting. Those who are more task oriented feel inhibited because work, progress, and change are evaluated only in terms of how they will affect others. A project to reorganize a reception area and rewrite job descriptions may be slowed and then stopped out of fear that the three employees in the area will be hurt by the change.

The Case of the Golden Lining The Cloudy Day Clinic had been through some tough times. Its much loved and esteemed if not autocratic, founder unexpectedly developed cancer and died. The clinic's staff were distressed about his death and were not prepared for a transition in leadership. An interim CEO, Dr. James, was quickly picked.

She was given the mission of holding down the fort and taking care of the staff, which she immediately set out to do. She met one-on-one with the entire staff and also developed a number of well-attended social occasions. She proceeded in her administrative work in a low-key manner that smoothed over problems and conflict. When difficult problems occurred or major decisions had to be made, she almost invariably got others involved and encouraged them to take on the tough problems and make the major or controversial decisions. During these times, she was always supportive and invariably adopted the recommendation of a committee or the advice of individuals willing to step forward to take charge. Gradually, the overarching lack of direction created some power struggles to get control of the decision-making process, which eventually compromised the clinic's ability to operate effectively.

Intervention Strategy The desire to take care of others and in return be taken care of is part of the give and take of life. However, when stress is great and self-esteem is diminished, some healthcare or physician executive's look to others to take charge. Anyone willing to lead during a stressful time is supported.

This executive can become difficult to deal with, in part, because he or she seems so nice and relatively innocent. It seems unfair to pressure this executive into making decisions and assuming personal responsibility. Employees intuitively know this and may discourage fellow employees from trying. Coaching and mentoring interventions by superiors can be approached as growth opportunities where the executive is expected to assume responsibility without being taken care of by others. Subordinates can also be successful if they are patient and persistent, waiting for the executive to own his or her responsibility rather than rushing in to assume it.

Dealing with this healthcare or physician executive's tendency to assume a dependent role requires acknowledging that rescuing the executive from his or her problems is a seductive fantasy. Care must be taken to coach the executive through a successful confrontation with the stressful situation even if initially there is considerable resistance and an excessive amount of time passes before he or she responds with the appropriate action. The resistance may include rejection and manipulation of the coaching executive, who must be willing to accept that it may take a long time before the dependent executive responds. This lengthy waiting period can create a lot of anxiety for the coaching executive. It is for this reason that care must be taken to select coaching situations where time is not of the essence.

For example, physicians often have considerable difficulty addressing performance issues. They are prone to submit positive staff evaluations and then suddenly complain about poor performance. Some physicians and physician executives are even willing to suffer through the poorest of performance rather than deal with a termination. In these circumstances, documenting complaints and patiently coaching the physician into making, if necessary, a truthful interim performance evaluation is the first step. If the more critical evaluation does not create progress, the physician may be coached into taking progressive disciplinary measures. It is not inappropriate for the clinic manager to become involved at this point, which to some extent externalizes the locus of control for the physician. However, external intervention will not be accepted by most physicians unless they are willing to recognize that a problem exists and that they can use some help resolving it. The medical group manager, a hospital and network executive, or another physician executive should be discouraged from coming in and solving the problem for the physician. This type of rescue blocks the physician executive's long-term development.

The Appeal to Freedom

Freedom is a word not often mentioned at work. Yet, employees may desire freedom from workplace pressure and freedom to work independently in order to function well in their job. Denial of such freedom can be harmful, but abuse of freedom can affect one's ability to cope with the many problems that work life presents. Personal goals and aspirations are often forfeited, as they require taking risks. These reclusive healthcare or physician executives seldom set personal goals or develop their ideas. They make it clear that they prefer to be left alone. In sum, unreasonable desire for a lack of supervision and participation in work life is unrealistic and detrimental to collaboration and group success.

The Resigned Leadership Style

The appeal to freedom results in the resigned leadership style. This healthcare or physician executive leadership style is sought out by network, hospital, and medical group members who prefer an inactive leader or someone who ignores the real world in favor of developing a stress-free workplace. This leader makes few demands of him- or herself and of others and limits anyone who advocates change. This healthcare or physician executive also minimizes conflict and usually resolves problems by taking the line of least resistance, including low-performance expectations, which may lead to low morale.

A typical example of this type of leadership is a hospital executive who, upon being assigned an important managerial role, accomplishes little and is opposed to oversight or receiving help. The area involved may be a testing laboratory, a particular product line, or a practice site. The executive wants to avoid the meddling interference of others and tends to create a group culture that is resistant to oversight from even the hospital's CEO. A hospital executive assigned the responsibility for managing a new and prospering practice site may, even after much coaching by the hospital's CEO, not accomplish the needed improvements and become openly resentful of being constantly pushed into making them.

Networks, hospitals, and medical groups may find the resigned leadership style suits certain aspects of their operation. For example, some types of work seem to attract people who prefer to be left alone to do their work. Production-oriented areas such as computing, pathology, and medical records may function best when left alone. Leaders of these types of areas will generally try to maintain this status. It is also possible that powerful department heads prefer a leader who will do little and leave them alone to pursue their own interests.

The Case of Misdirection The Blue Skies Health Center, after a few years of operation, reached a point in its development where a major reorganization was needed to address many unresolved issues surrounding its rapid growth. The center had been well received, and many specialists had been rapidly added. Their practices flourished, which led to further expansion of specialization, the development of subspecialty services, the development of contracts with managed care organizations, and the acquisition of preferred provider status with several major employers.

The dynamic growth required a corporate-like management structure, and a new structure was agreed to with the assistance of a consultant. The new structure required the selection of a CEO. The center director ruled himself out as a candidate.

An extensive search ensued with the help of a search firm. The search firm initially interviewed all of the department heads and learned that they wanted a dynamic, well-organized, visionary leader to lead continued growth of the center. A number of good candidates were located and interviewed, but none were found acceptable. The search firm's representative was puzzled by this outcome, as a number of the candidates were outstanding leaders. A second round of candidates yielded similar results.

It was at this point that a candidate was put forward by several of the department heads. This individual was less qualified and, in fact, had a track record of accomplishing little in a role where much could have been done.

Mr. Dolittle received a positive response from many of the department heads, and the decision was made to offer him the CEO position. Despite the fact that this was baffling to the search firm's representative, Mr. Dolittle was hired and the medical staff and key managers were happy. It was clear to the search firm's representative that the department heads, while verbalizing a desire for strong leadership, enjoyed their autonomy and feared that the hiring of an experienced medical group executive would undermine their power. As a result of Mr. Dolittle's complacency and unwillingness to set direction, coordinate, or resolve conflict, Blue Skies gradually became uncompetitive because of its poor problem-solving ability.

Intervention Strategy The desire to be left alone to do whatever you want is as natural as any of the other appeals. However, this tendency may also become an extreme where interactions with others and task assignments are experienced as coercive and controlling and, therefore, to be avoided. The result may be an executive who is resistant to supervision, taking direction, setting goals, and working with others. This healthcare or physician executive is also more than willing to leave others alone and avoids having to give direction to or set goals for others, as was the case for Mr. Dolittle and the leaders of the Blue Skies Health Center who also wanted to be left alone.

Dealing with a healthcare or physician executive who frequently retreats from interaction and who has problems setting goals for self and others requires patience and persistence. Confrontation will be experienced as threatening and coercive. Superiors will have as much difficulty as subordinates in being effective in dealing with this executive. Instructions, requests, questions, feedback, and direct orders are all negative influences that the executive prefers to avoid, and passive expressions of aggression may abound. It is important to approach the executive firmly but not in such way as to promote defensiveness. It should be made clear that the executive must be prepared to meet performance criteria and receive feedback without retreating from the interaction. Subordinates must be equally persistent and appreciate that their assuming this executive's responsibility can also lead to double binds with the executive who may prefer no one take any action. Coaching will involve working with the healthcare or physician executive to set goals, followed by a watchful eye as they are carried out. Stressful conditions will usually aggravate this psychologically defensive tendency, which may gradually lead to passive resistance and aggression and work being assigned to others. This has the effect of fulfilling this executive's unconscious interpersonal agenda of avoidance. Tendencies to work around this executive must be avoided if the executive is to learn to be more willing to accept direction and goal setting.

In summary, a resigned network, hospital, or physician executive who is suspicious and resentful of oversight and interventions made by others may feel that demands are being made and that the expectations being placed on him or her are coercive. As a result, this executive may feel justified in fending them off. Interventions must first begin with this appreciation. They must also include a careful analysis of the situation, including data collection and analysis to be certain how work is being affected. Information may also be collected about those who work with the executive to determine if they have assumed the same attitude as their leader. Eventually, the resigned executive must be confronted with the carefully developed data, and he or she must be coached into setting firm goals and time boundaries. If this approach is resisted, it may be prudent to make a change in leadership. If the approach is accepted, progress must be documented and discussed at suitable periods. Some of these executives may eventually recognize they just do not like the responsibility and will resign. Others may be pushed into a period of personal development where they overcome their psychologically defensive tendency and become productive leaders.

Contemporary Leadership Styles Compared to the Psychologically Defensive Leadership Styles

Thus far, this chapter has introduced a new psychologically informed typology of executive leadership styles. These styles arise from deeply held and often unconscious motivations. They also contribute to better understanding traditional contemporary typologies of leadership.

There are many additional ways to understand leadership and leadership styles. Some common ones are highlighted below. These styles of leadership have been, for the most part, developed from observing or interviewing leaders. These typologies are informative and are the grist of countless management courses. However, what is important to appreciate is that they do not explain the psychological origins of leadership behavior. Understanding a leader's thoughts and feelings is critical to gaining a true appreciation of what motivates his or her behavior. The above five psychologically defensive leadership styles and the intentional leadership style do address the psychological side of leadership, and it is possible to match the following traditional typologies to the psychologically defensive leadership styles.

Gordon L. Lippitt classifies leadership based upon decision-making styles.[3]

- *Autocratic* decision makers make all of the decisions and pass them down to subordinates.
- *Laissez-faire* decision makers leave decision making to their subordinates.
- *Democratic* decision makers permit employees to participate in decisions.
- *Benevolent autocratic* decision makers make the decisions but only after consultation with subordinates.

George R. Terry and R.H. Hermanson classify leadership by the type of organizational communication and interaction the leader uses.[4]

- *Personal* leadership involves the leader developing friendships with subordinates using face-to-face communication.
- *Nonpersonal* leadership involves subordinates communicating among themselves and reliance upon oaths and pledges to create conforming behavior.
- *Democratic* leadership involves open discussion and participation in decision making.
- *Paternalistic* leadership involves the leader encouraging dependence by withholding decision-making authority and resources and assuming the role of protector of members of the organization.

- *Authoritarian* leadership involves the leader making all of the decisions based upon formal organizational power and authority.
- *Indigenous* leadership involves others, as needed and from time to time, providing leadership when the formal leader is present.

Glenn A. Bassett describes leadership in terms of its long-term effects upon organizational culture.[5]

- The *authoritarian* leader makes all of the decisions, provides all of the organization's values, discourages individual initiative, and promotes dependence.
- The *permissive* leader does not take an active part in decision making or the setting of organizational values. This promotes employee independence, initiative, self-development, and the assumption of significant responsibility for the organization's operation.
- The *integrative* leader is neither authoritarian nor permissive and encourages open participation under his or her direction.

Stephen J. Knezevich classifies leadership by using descriptive terms that contain positive and negative connotations.[6]

- The *autocratic* leader makes all of the decisions.
- The *democratic* leader allows participation in decision making.
- The *anarchic* leader provides no direction; employees run the organization.
- The *manipulative* or *pseudodemocratic* leader makes all of the decisions but then appoints committees to endorse them to give the appearance of participation.

J. W. Getzels and E.G. Guba provide a leadership continuum where two of the classifications are at either end and a third is at the mid-point.[7]

- *Nomothetic* leaders desire unthinking compliance and impose rules and formal organization roles to enforce conformity.
- *Idiographic* leaders delegate and encourage the meeting of individual needs and goals over those of the organization.
- *Transactional* leaders balance employee and organizational interests but may adopt one of the above two leadership styles depending upon the circumstances.

William J. Reddin classifies leadership according to its effectiveness as measured by the fit between task-oriented and relationship-oriented leadership styles and the situation of the moment.[8] For example, a relationship-oriented, low-task leadership style may be effective in a care giving organization but ineffective in a factory. The following styles of leadership are usually ineffective under most circumstances:

- The *autocratic* high-task and low-interpersonal style makes it clear that the leader does not trust others.
- The *missionary* low-task and high-interpersonal style sacrifices organizational effectiveness to promote harmony.
- The *deserter* low-task and low-interpersonal style is uninvolved, avoids interpersonal contact, and provides little leadership or direction.

The following leadership styles are usually more effective but must be employed in a manner that is consistent with the work or problem at hand:

- The *executive* high-task and high-interpersonal style provides motivation by providing clear direction, setting meaningful performance standards, and treating employees according to their individual needs.
- The *benevolent dictator* high-task and low-interpersonal style fulfills his or her goals while not alienating others.

- The *developer* low-task and high-interpersonal style trusts others and is interested in their well-being.
- The *bureaucrat* low-task and low-interpersonal style uses rules and procedures to enforce conformity in pursuit of organizational goals.

Alexander W. Astin and Rita A. Scherrei provide five classifications for leaders:[9]

- *Hierarchical* leaders communicate little, reward competitiveness, discourage openness and critical thinking, and frustrate needs for recognition and security.
- *Humanist* leaders permit open communication, reward openness and critical thinking, discourage competitiveness and rivalry, and create a comfortable workplace setting.
- *Entrepreneurial* leaders are aggressive, risk taking, competitive, and frank and reward these attributes in others.
- *Insecure* leaders reward "apple polishing," influence peddling, and cronyism, discourage creativity and risk taking, and tend to create an atmosphere filled with gossip and manipulative behavior.
- *Task-oriented* leaders encourage initiative, cooperation, and competence and usually create a work setting where employees feel secure and valued.

Physician Executive Leadership Styles

A study by Jensen involving 45 two-hour interviews of physician executives resulted in the description of five types of physician executive leadership styles.[10] These five leadership patterns each have their own management philosophy, approaches to work, and ways of relating to external groups.

The *practice physician* executive believes in rational problem solving as the best way to manage the medical group. Problems are to be analyzed, alternatives developed, and optimal choices made. This physician executive possesses humanistic values and is concerned with developing stability, cooperation, and harmony within the medical group. He or she believes that demonstrated needs should be funded and that persistent pressure combined with rational argument promotes change. This physician has a cooperative attitude toward external groups, which he or she believes are potential patient care resources, and he or she believes that physicians are artisans who should be supported by their medical group.

The *professional physician* executive also believes that the medical group should provide a stable and supportive structure for patient care. This physician executive, however, believes that organizational norms do not apply to physicians who seek excellence and that healthcare organizations do not need to conform to social norms. This executive willingly assumes responsibility and leadership roles. He or she strives for excellence, and others are expected to work in a professional manner. This physician also feels that external groups threaten his or her and the medical group's autonomy. Outsiders are expected to learn that the medical group is unique and that the positions of its leaders are correct. This executive strives for an aristocratic image and to differentiate him- or herself from other physicians in terms of importance. He or she is only willing to work with others if they are working on a task judged to be desirable.

The *self-physician* executive sees the medical group as a battle field for getting his or her way. Victories and defeats are felt to be temporary. There are always more battles left to be waged. This physician executive seeks control over work and employees, must know what everyone is doing, wants to make all of the decisions, and is willing to manipulate others to win. This physician is also adept at relating to others who control external groups and believes that the norms and values of others do not apply to him or her. He or she is willing to attack external groups to fulfill his or her aims and enjoys battles, seeing them as a way to improve him- or herself and the medical group.

The *organizational physician* executive approaches work differently. This physician executive believes that the medical group can achieve it ends through scientific management and rational structuring of the group, work, and decision making. The team approach is stressed. Everyone is expected to contribute, and no one area is permitted to outgrow another. This physician approaches work from the point of view that personal and medical group responsibilities should be kept separate. This physician is willing to devote large amounts of time to making the medical group succeed and encourages others to participate. Relations with external groups are governed by a competitive response. This competitive leader develops an image of a capitalist and entrepreneur who is paving the way for the success of his or her medical group. This is, in part, accomplished by hiring outstanding performers to enhance the medical group's competitive edge.

The *syntonic physician* executive believes that the medical group needs a leader who is willing to take risks and make enemies, project the future, inspire others to excel, assume leadership roles, work hard, and make the tough decisions. This executive supports others and accepts individual and situational limitations. He or she approaches work from the point of view of keeping others focused on their assigned work and tries to resolve differences of opinion without feeling the need to take charge and control everything. He or she permits open and direct exchanges, seeks dialogue and promotes solutions to conflicts by emphasizing interrelatedness. He or she seeks to project an image of wisdom and balance and thinks of him- or herself as someone who is able to deal with stress, diversity, and multiple issues without becoming distressed.

Jensen believes that physician executives vacillate between the more balanced (syntonic) leadership style—which takes into consideration aspects of the other four leadership patterns—and the four less desirable leadership patterns. It is also worth noting that these different leadership styles share much in common with and are in many ways explained by the psychologically defensive leadership styles discussed in this chapter. These relationships will subsequently be pointed out.

These authors have consistently located similar content in their observations of leadership behavior. It is also obvious that these leadership styles abound in networks, hospitals, and medical groups. Healthcare and physician executives must also appreciate that leadership styles are influenced by issues related to interpersonal power and authority and to personal needs to feel autonomous, liked, and admired. Dealing with or changing leadership style is, therefore, much more difficult than merely observing and classifying behavior. It must be appreciated that leadership style is based in personality and its accompanying but not so readily acknowledged unconscious and irrational elements.

Understanding the difference between lists of leadership characteristics and the underlying motivations for the development of the leadership styles is critical for better appreciating the true complexity of dealing with leaders. The intentional leadership style and each of the psychologically defensive leadership styles can be matched to the list of contemporary leadership characteristics first mentioned. By so doing, it will become clear that understanding leadership styles must involve understanding their underlying psychological defensive nature, which arises when stress increases and excessive anxiety is experienced.

The *appeal to mastery* and its three accompanying leadership styles (perfectionist, arrogant-vindictive, and narcissistic) may be grouped with the autocratic, benevolent dictator, manipulative or pseudodemocratic, authoritarian, paternalistic, nomothetic, bureaucratic, hierarchical, entrepreneurial, and the professional and self-physician leadership styles. The *appeal to love* and its accompanying self-effacing leadership style may be matched to benevolent autocrat, personal, idiographic, missionary, developer, humanistic, insecure, and practice physician leadership styles. The *appeal to freedom* and its accompanying resigned leadership style may be compared to the laissez-faire, anarchic, nonpersonal, and deserter leadership styles. By comparison, an intentional leadership style is matched to democratic, indigenous, integrative, transactional, executive, task-oriented, and organizational and syntonic leadership styles.

Conclusion

This chapter has examined leadership from the perspective that it may, from time to time, become less than intentional. Leadership is a complex concept. Many insights can be gained when the behavior of healthcare executives is scrutinized for psychologically defensive, self-protective tendencies. Many healthcare or physician executives unintentionally adopt psychologically defensive leadership styles when they find themselves experiencing excessive stress. Understanding one's own tendencies to adopt defensive leadership styles and the tendencies of others to adopt them is an important first step in being able to work effectively with the many executives of many organizations that must be combined to create large fully integrated regional healthcare delivery networks. Organizational performance can be improved by minimizing the need for self-protection by making the workplace less threatening and anxiety ridden. This can only occur, however, through the development of a supportive and open workplace, where both executives and employees can feel secure in learning self-reflective and interpretive skills. The outcome of this learning, while not changing personalities, does lead employees toward nondefensive interpretations of events and administrative actions.

Endnotes

1. Diamond, M. *The Unconscious Life of Organizations: Interpreting Organizational Identity.* Westport, Connecticut: Quorum, 1993.

2. The psychodynamic model in Figure 5 and its explanation are based upon the work of Michael A. Diamond and Seth

Allcorn, "Psychological Barriers to Personal Responsibility," *Organizational Dynamics* 12 (1984): 66–77; Michael A. Diamond and Seth Allcorn, "Psychological Responses to Stress in Complex Organizations," *Administration and Society* 17 (August 1985): 217–239; Michael A. Diamond and Seth Allcorn, "The Freudian Factor," *Personnel Journal* 69 (March 1990): 52–65; and Seth Allcorn, "Leadership Styles: The Psychological Picture," *Personnel* 65 (April 1988): 46–54. This work is based upon the psychoanalytic theory of Karen Horney who published *Neurosis and Human Growth* (New York: Norton, 1950).

3. G. L Lippitt, *Organizational Renewal* (Englewood Cliffs, New Jersey: Prentice-Hall, 1969).

4. G. R. Terry and R. H. Hermanson, *Principles of Management* (Homewood, IL: Learning Systems Co., 1970).

5. G. A. Basset, *Management Styles in Transition* (New York: American Management Association, 1966).

6. S. J. Knezevich, *Administration of Public Education* (New York: Harper & Row, 1969).

7. C. A. Getzels and E. G. Guba, "Social Behavior and the Administrative Process," *School Review* 65 (Winter 1957): 423–41.

8. W. J. Reddin, *Managerial Effectiveness* (New York: McGraw-Hill, 1970).

9. A. W. Aslin and R. A. Scherrei, *Maximizing Leadership Effectiveness* (San Francisco: Jossey-Bass, 1980).

10. A. T. Jensen, "Physician Executive Leadership," *Medical Group Management* 33 (September/October 1986): 20–30.

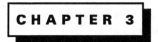

CHAPTER 3

UNDERSTANDING
DEFENSIVE DYNAMICS

The complexity of the interpersonal arena makes it important to have a conceptual scheme that can be used to understand often unconsciously motivated, psychologically defensive interpersonal dynamics. Psychological defensiveness and self-protective behavior (discussed in Chapter 2) are acted out in the interpersonal world. This eventuality makes examining the interaction of the psychologically defensive types important. There are twenty-one psychologically defensive interactions.[1] Figure 6 illustrates the defensive interactions explained in this chapter. The defensive types are listed along both axes of the diagram or matrix, and the Xs are placed in the cells to be discussed. In order to gain an appreciation of the significance of the interactions, each marked cell in Figure 6 is described as though two executives of different healthcare organizations are interacting either over developing an integrated arrangement or over change that must occur after integration.

I have used for my examples healthcare and physician executives below the level of chief executive officer (CEO). These positions include chief financial officer (CFO), chief information officer (CIO), chief operating officer (COO), human resources executives, legal counsel, and the many subordinates to these roles. They are referred to in the generic sense—executives—to avoid referring to them with longer expressions such as healthcare and physician executives or CEO/CFO. It must also be noted that the other unmarked cells of the matrix could also be discussed. They reverse the interpersonal encounters described in this chapter and

Figure 6   Matrix of Interpersonal Psychological Defensiveness

	PERFECTIONIST	ARROGANT-VINDICTIVE	NARCISSIST	SELF-EFFACING	RESIGNED	INTENTIONAL
PERFECTIONIST	X					
ARROGANT-VINDICTIVE	X	X				
NARCISSIST	X	X	X			
SELF-EFFACING	X	X	X	X		
RESIGNED	X	X	X	X	X	
INTENTIONAL	X	X	X	X	X	X

the next. They are, however, not discussed as they add little additional insight for the amount of additional reading involved.

The interventions suggested are, in all cases, described as though a CEO of a network is making them. Given that senior level executives are involved in the negotiations and subsequent management of the integrated organization, the network CEO is the individual who can most appropriately and successfully intervene in the dysfunctional interpersonal dynamics discussed. However, the suggested intervention strategies can also be applied by the CEOs of other organizations within the network and executives below the level of CEO when those involved in dysfunctional behavior are below them in the organizational hierarchy of the network, hospital, or medical group. It must also be acknowledged that colleagues and friends can successfully intervene given the right circumstances. Finally, it is also possible for an executive who finds him- or herself paired with an anxious and defensive colleague or negotiator from another organization to intervene in the dysfunctional interpersonal dynamics. Therefore, intervention is not limited to the top-down variety. Not to be overlooked are interventions made by in-house group process consultants or external consultants who are trained to facilitate change. These consultants can be effective in creating collaboration by confronting and working through dysfunctional executive psychological defensiveness. This chapter, however, focuses on intervention by CEOs or other senior level executives to simplify discussion and because they are very likely the most common sources of interventions.

Many who have read the psychologically defensive types have identified superiors, friends, and colleagues. These realizations are important and should be used to promote learning and reflection. At the same time, care must be taken to avoid labeling others based upon the types discussed. People are more complex than just one type and will often act out more than one psychologically defensive strategy depending on the reactions of others even though one strategy may be much more frequently relied on. Labeling may, therefore, blind the observer to seeing changes in the psychological defensive strategy being used or the emergence of a blend of strategies. It is also important to keep in mind our own psychologically defensive tendencies, which affect how we respond to stress and the defensive tendencies of others. It is important to try to remain self-reflective in order to be able to spot defensive changes in one's own thoughts, feelings, and actions.

It must also be appreciated that observing the interactions of others leads to considering how to intervene in interpersonally defensive and unproductive working relationships. An intervention strategy is briefly described after each dysfunctional interaction is explained. Interventions must be carefully timed and well considered, and they should not provoke more anxiety and defensiveness.

The role of the intervening individual is also an important aspect of the intervention. Interventions may involve direct discussion of the behavior observed, which might be the case if a CEO, process consultant, or trusted colleague or friend makes the intervention. Less empowered interventions by colleagues and fellow negotiators have to rely on a constant press of coaching and suggestions to redirect energy from psychologically defensive strategies to ones that are more intentional and productive for the network. There are no easy answers as to exactly how to intervene in the dysfunctional psychologically defensive behavior of senior level executives. There is no cookbook, two-minute approach to helping these executives become more effective at working together under the stressful conditions of constant change. All senior level executives have had to coach, counsel, prod, train, encourage, and even occasionally insist that one or more executives under their direction change their work process and the methods and nature of their interactions to achieve less conflicted, competitive, and power- and control-oriented behavior. How this is accomplished depends on the people involved, the situation, and moment.

Therefore, the interventions discussed below are phrased in broad terms intended to guide critical thinking about how to approach and change the organizationally dysfunctional, psychologically defensive behavior of the executives involved. In sum, understanding the interpersonal situation in terms of the interactions discussed will empower executives with a better understanding of what is going on and why, which leads to more insightful interventions on their part. My experience as a healthcare executive has proven to me that successful interventions are possible.

I now turn to the discussion of the pairs of psychologically defensive types. Discussing the pairs of interactions provides an opportunity to explore the many complexities of interpersonal relationships in a systematic manner. These 21 types of interactions occur often enough in the healthcare workplace to merit discussion of each.

Perfectionist versus Perfectionist

These executives compete by setting rigorous standards for each other to meet, which leads to a proliferation of unrealistic performance criteria. This competitive standard setting process leads them to constantly judge and criticize each other, the work process, the products of their work, and the other's organization and staff. Each strives to be more perfect than the other, which limits collaboration and leads to excessive attention on unproductive and tedious detail. This is exhausting for all concerned. Negotiations to purchase the assets of a medical group may, for example, become bogged down in efforts to think through every eventuality, to develop ever more accurate appraisals, and to further perfect the wording of the legal agreement. Neither executive seems able to be pleased in all respects, and neither is willing to back off.

Intervention Strategy

An intervention by the network CEO must focus on limiting the pursuit of perfection by these executives in favor of their making some compromises. These executives must be allowed to feel it is acceptable to hold high standards; however, when they use the standards to be critical of each other, they must be encouraged to stay on task and avoid attacking each other. A firm hand is needed to avoid their tendency to try to control each other by being excessively critical. They must also be reminded that accomplishing the task within an acceptable time limit is important and that constantly nitpicking and obsessing over every detail is counterproductive. They must also be reminded that some aspects of the work can be resolved after an agreement or operating change is made.

A network CEO, when confronted with two team leaders who are constantly criticizing each other in meetings, in correspondence, and directly to the CEO, decides to meet with each separately and then with both together. During the individual meetings, the CEO reviews each executive's point of view and reasons for the point of view. In each case, overly perfectionistic aspects of their positions are uncovered and discussed for what they are, overly perfectionistic, which is promoting conflict and blocking work. At the same time, their work and values are applauded as delivering a good final product. After an open and frank discussion with each, the CEO asks them to jointly meet with him to review where they are in their work and what their differences of opinion are. The CEO works with the two in an open and collaborative mode to resolve these differences and occasionally makes a decision that resolves an unresolved problem. The meeting concludes with a review of the importance of collaboration.

Perfectionist versus Arrogant-Vindictive

The perfectionist executive is frequently critical and offends the arrogant-vindictive executive's sensitive pride. In return, the arrogant-vindictive executive counterattacks and tries to dominate and outcompete his or her critical counterpart. The inevitable outcome is a combative working relationship that produces unpredictable outcomes as each executive tries to control the other and his or her anxiety. The perfectionist finds it easy to criticize his or her arrogant-vindictive counterpart who often seems indifferent to what others think and feel. In return, the arrogant-vindictive executive holds a lot of contempt for the perfectionist who never seems to get anything done, who is always buzzing around with criticism, and who never really comes out to fight. An example is the closing of a redundant lab in the perfectionist's hospital, which may lead to interminable discussions of what will happen to the employees, space, patients, physicians, and so on, which will inevitably infuriate the arrogant-vindictive executive who is trying to expeditiously accomplish the closing on behalf of the network.

The network executive eventually explodes in a meeting, pounding the table angrily and yelling at the hospital executive who it is explained is dragging his feet. The hospital executive's response is to again explain all of his points, an explanation which is rudely interrupted. At this point, he says no more, folds up his papers, and appears ready to leave. The network executive, having vented his rage, is also ready to end the meeting. Both leave, and nothing is accomplished. Each retreats to his superior to complain about the other's behavior.

Intervention Strategy

This is a challenging intervention for any CEO. If these two executives can be kept on task, they accomplish good work. The perfectionist contributes an attention to detail and high standards, while the arrogant-vindictive executive can be effective at leading the charge to get a change implemented. In the above scenerio, a division of duties may work where the perfectionist is encouraged to focus on developing the plans and the arrogant-vindictive executive is asked to expend his energy on overcoming problems of implementation. This approach builds on the strengths of each and will tend to minimize the always present and potentially destructive nature of their interpersonal psychologically defensive tendencies.

Due to the importance of getting the redundant lab closed, the network CEO decides to meet with his executive and the hospital lab manager after clearing the meeting with the laboratory manager's superior. The meeting with the lab manager focuses on understanding many of his major points and locating areas where excessive perfection is being expected from the change process. These areas are further explored, and the CEO, while understanding the manager's concern, asks that many of them be dropped for now in favor of moving ahead. The manager's feelings are taken into account by acknowledging the lab's contribution thus far to the network and the sad but necessary closing at this point.

The meeting with his network executive focuses on his tendency to blow up at times and his feelings of constantly being in a war zone where winning becomes the only thing that matters. At the same time the behavior of the perfectionist laboratory manager is explored as something he does not easily tolerate. The CEO points out that it is important to respect the perfectionist's basic tendencies and challenge only those that are excessively perfectionistic, critical, and overcontrolling. He is then asked to meet with the laboratory manager and to begin the meeting by apologizing for his outburst. He is also told that the CEO believes that the lab manager will back off on his concerns and demands in a number of areas in order to close the lab. The CEO asks him to call him after their meeting to provide an overview of what was agreed to and how well they were able to work together.

Perfectionist versus Narcissist

The perfectionist executive seeks to impose many restrictive and hard-to-meet standards on the working relation. The promulgation of the standards is accompanied by a tireless attention to detail and frequent criticism. The narcissistic executive may try to meet some of the standards to receive approval that cannot ultimately be obtained. At the same time, the narcissist has little patience for details and prefers to work with the big picture, which infuriates the perfectionist. Their working relationship will be periodically tense as the narcissist moves toward fulfilling a big idea that gets bogged down in all the details that the perfectionist introduces into the relationship. These two executives, however, tend to provide balance for each other; if they succeed in producing an outcome, it may be a good idea that is reasonably well thought through and documented. For example, a negotiation for the purchase of the assets of a long-term care facility may take much longer than the narcissistic network executive prefers, but the purchase agreement may be one that is quite serviceable once it is hammered out. On the other hand, the negotiations may collapse as the long-term care facility's perfectionist executive seeks ever-greater control to combat anxiety, and the narcissistic network executive gives up trying to receive approval and wants to move onto another big project.

For example, a network CFO is confronted with an intractable negotiation to an already agreed to purchase of a long-term care facility. Investigation by the CEO reveals that despite clear direction from the facility's board to arrange the sale, the manager of the facility is pursuing a strategy of trying to wring out every last dime in the sale by generating volumes of information and contracting with outside accessors to place a high value on the facility and its equipment. The network CFO has just about given up trying to deal with the manager and has begun to focus his energies on a new, more exciting project. This has left a vacuum where progress toward arranging the sale has been slowed to a crawl. An intervention by the network CEO is in order.

Intervention Strategy

This intervention is also demanding for the network CEO as each executive has tendencies that frustrate the other's unconscious desires. The narcissist is the dreamer with big ideas who seeks attention, approval, and admiration from others. The perfectionist tends to work in the background, always trying to improve agreements and operations. The perfectionist is also not a particularly creative person and seldom develops grand visions, which are, it is unconsciously felt, too difficult to perfect anyway. In sum, the narcissist introduces an important aspect of creativity and vision into the relationship that the perfectionist can be encouraged to build upon and perfect. They may, however, both be weak on implementation where excessive attention to detail or lack of appreciation of detail can become an inhibitor. Simi-

71

larly, implementation of change often requires forceful and effective leadership, something the narcissist may avoid because of conflict and the fear of loss of admiration and the perfectionist may compromise by being constantly critical and unrewarding. CEOs must be on the lookout for these tendencies.

In the above example, the network CEO intervened by meeting with both executives separately. The meeting with the manger of the long-term facility began with a view of information about the sale of the facility to the network. The manager was asked to confirm the information, and misunderstandings were discussed. The manager was then asked to review her progress in arranging the sale, and instances where measures were excessive and perfectionistic were discussed. Agreement was eventually reached as to the final steps to be taken and an approximate time frame for their accomplishment. The meeting with the network executive responsible for arranging the purchase revealed that he had lost interest in dealing with the manager, who obsessed over everything and seemed resistant and passive-aggressive. The CEO communicated that his meeting with the manager went well and that she seemed prepared to finish the work in an orderly, timely, and not overly controlling manner. The network CFO was asked to resume work on the purchase arrangements and to keep the CEO informed via biweekly progress reports.

Perfectionist versus Self-Effacing

These executives find themselves to be more alike than different The self-effacing executive holds perfectionistic self-expectations that cannot be met which creates feelings of worthlessness, helpless, and deficiency. He or she is never good enough. The perfectionist executive constantly reinforces these tendencies to feel worthless and deficient by promulgating hard-to-meet standards, paying close attention to details, and offering frequent criticism. The admiring and dependent self-effacing executive looks up to the judgmental perfectionist, which flatters and reinforces the perfectionist in his or her pursuit of interpersonal control through perfection. Both executives will very likely believe everything will turn out right if the perfectionist succeeds. At the same time, the self-effacing executives needs to be taken care of by a powerful other who is admired and even loved in return.

A self-effacing executive who needs to change and strengthen a home infusion service may eagerly accept direction from a perfectionist network executive who appears to want to achieve the highest of standards for the service and who seems to know exactly how it needs to be changed and is not afraid to say so. This executive who has prior experience setting up and operating home infusion services and is authoritative about what to do also, at times, denigrates his colleague and the employees of the service. However, his many unilateral interventions are welcomed by the home infusion program executive, and the staff are cooperative. As a result, much rapid change is made, some of which takes on excessive proportions as unrealistic performance and control criteria are eventually set. However, the infusion executive accepts the standards and constant criticism without complaint and usually feels thankful that the network executive is there to help run the service at least for now. However, employees of the service begin to eventually complain to anyone who will listen.

Intervention Strategy

These two executives will usually work well together as a result of reinforcing each other's psychologically defensive interpersonal strategy. The relationship can be improved by discouraging the perfectionist from being constantly critical of his or her self-effacing counterpart who is willing to suffer humiliation in order to remain attached and dependent. If the perfectionist has tendencies to take out his or her feelings on others by being critical, this potentially sadistic tendency needs to be minimized. The perfectionist can be encouraged to assume a mentoring role that includes helping his or her colleague to become more independent rather than less. In contrast, the self-effacing executive needs to be encouraged to feel that he or she is capable of functioning without the constant direction of the perfectionist, and he or she must be discouraged from constant self-criticism, self-minimization, and masochistic tendencies.

In the above example, employee complaints increased as they felt they were being over controlled and monitored, and constantly criticized and micromanaged by the network executive with the tacit consent of their boss. The CEO eventually intervened to discuss the situation individually with the two executives and then with them together. He also wanted to know if staff development were occurring so that the amount of micromanagment would diminish. He reported that it seemed necessary because the infusion service manager was fairly passive and not proactive. The network executive was reminded that it was important to try to develop the manager's talents and that by constantly intervening, he was promoting dependency and a lack of development on the part of the infusion service manager. Also discussed were the many performance standards that had been developed and whether some of them expected too much and would invariably result in failure and criticism, which was adversely affecting employee morale. The executive agreed to reconsider the standards with an eye towards what was realistic. The meeting with the service manager focused on developing a more active, take-charge leadership style and on how the CEO and the network could help the manager with this important developmental work. Leadership training was agreed to. The joint meeting yielded a meeting of the minds as the network executive had already adjusted the standards and was beginning to assume more responsibility as a result of feeling supported by the executive, CEO and network.

Perfectionist versus Resigned

The ever-busy and critical perfectionist is experienced by the resigned executive as excessively judgmental, self-centered, and invasive. Interpersonal boundaries are vigorously defended by the resigned executive, who makes every effort to avoid the perfectionist and his or her criticism. The perfectionist will, however, pursue the retreating resigned executive, who is easily criticized for not being a contributor and who never seems to stand up for him- or herself. The result is two people who can not easily work together and very likely cannot produce anything of value. The perfectionist dominates the relationship, and the resigned executive may eventually agree to anything, thereby underrepresenting his or her interests, staff, and organization.

Negotiations to purchase a rehabilitation service will be dominated by a perfectionist who, on behalf of the network, eagerly develops draft after draft of the purchase agreement only to find that the rehabilitation service's resigned executive responsible for completing the negotiations is rather indifferent to all of the paperwork and willing to essentially sacrifice the development of a better deal for the service's current owners and employees rather than become actively involved in dealing with the perfectionist. This outcome, of course, creates a win-lose outcome that is beneficial to the network; however, the owners of the service reject most of the plan for purchase, thereby creating a timing crisis and the need to start over with the negotiations.

Intervention Strategy

These two psychologically defensive interpersonal tendencies are like the poles of two magnets, they inherently push themselves apart. The perfectionist is eager to try to take control and dominate, and the resigned executive is just as eager to avoid being dominated and coerced into meeting standards, deadlines, and goals. The harder the perfectionist pushes, the more resistant and unavailable the resigned executive becomes. Intervening in these interpersonal dynamics is challenging. The

75

perfectionist's tendencies must be minimized, while the resigned executive's tendency to withdraw must be addressed by trying to draw him or her into a working relationship with the perfectionist that promises not to be too interpersonally invasive and critical.

In the above example, the network CEO intervened with the approval of the service's owners. A meeting with the executive of the service revealed a person who was not assertive and avoided interacting with the CEO over the issues surrounding the purchase. The CEO, using information about the executive's behavior exhibited in the meeting, raised the issue that in order for the work to be accomplished, everyone needed her participation and input, which was important to both the owners and the network as a fair deal was the goal. She agreed that she would commit herself to learning what the owners wanted from the sale and try to effectively represent their interests in the negotiations. The meeting with the network executive focused on his need to back off a bit and to avoid dominating the manager and the negotiations, which had played a role in creating an unacceptable purchase agreement. The executive was encouraged to help the manager represent the owner's interests effectively while not necessarily agreeing to everything. He had to take the position of trying to develop a fair deal even though the service's manager had a tendency to give up too easily.

Perfectionist versus Intentionalist

Perfectionist executives attempt to impose standards on their intentional colleagues, who will sometimes agree to them and try to meet them and at other times reject them or seek to modify them. As a result, the development of perfectionistic standards and criticism does not consistently have the hoped-for effect on the intentional executive (that of controlling the executive), which can be frustrating to the perfectionist. The intentional executive finds the perfectionistic executive occasionally difficult to work with and preoccupied with perfectionism, detail, and control, which inhibits progress.

A perfectionist network executive who seeks to change an ambulatory program of a large, multispecialty group by removing expensive testing and therapeutic equipment duplicated elsewhere in the network will not always find his or her intentional medical group colleague willing to acknowledge the perfectionist's ideas as better or even appropriate. However, some of them are accepted (intermittent reinforcement), which encourages greater efforts by the perfectionist to develop more standards and detailed proposals and plans. In return, the intentionalist avoids becoming distressed with the perfectionist's behavior even though it is at times overly demanding. The negotiations, however, progress at a reasonable pace and do not become bogged down in detail, although the network executive is occasionally angry at and critical of the medical group's executive. There is however, give-and-take in the discussions.

Intervention Strategy

Network CEOs who observe this interaction will spot the presence of an intentionalist by his or her balanced approach to work. His or her nondefensive tendencies must be encouraged. At the same time, the perfectionist must be encouraged to be less defensive and controlling and, therefore, perfectionistic and critical. His or her attention must be directed to finding a workable solution rather than a perfect one.

The CEO, during a meeting with the above two executives, observes that the network executive has developed a number of comprehensive and exacting analyses and proposals and periodically dominates the meeting with them as well as occasionally criticizing others including the medical group manager who does not appear to take much offense. The medical group manager provides thoughtful feedback on the network executive's discussion, analyses and, proposals, while offering several of her own. As the meeting proceeds, the CEO gradually begins to focus on some of the more extreme points, positions, and standards put forward by the network executive and, while acknowledging that it is important to achieve excellence in the work, it is also noted that there are times when it is appropriate to accept a little less than perfection in making a change and that in order to expedite the change, some compromise with the medical group manager's point of view is necessary.

Arrogant-Vindictive versus Arrogant-Vindictive

These two executives find themselves locked in a struggle for dominance and control. Each is ultimately out to eliminate the other. Each is suspicious of the other and believes that he or she is out to get him or her. Their untrusting and competitive interactions tend to reinforce these beliefs. Accomplishing the task at hand is subordinated to the struggle for dominance, although each individual may become productive in the process of trying to outperform the other by working harder and taking more risks.

Negotiations or working relationships that require cooperation are compromised by these two executives, who are often unyielding in defending their point of view and more than willing to constantly attack the other's point of view. Little work may be accomplished unless one ends up dominating the other, which vindicates his or her arrogant pride and may result in the ruthless subordination of the loser who feared this outcome and who will be ready to strike back at the first opportunity. Discussions as to how to best optimize a hospital's productivity may become hopelessly deadlocked, and there may not appear to be any way to salvage the situation.

For example, the managers of the gastroenterology service and the surgical service, when asked to merge their endoscopy and colonoscopy labs, almost immediately reached many impasses in working out the merger. The physicians and staff involved became equally concerned about their lab being taken over by the other department rather than a new third department.

Intervention Strategy

Intervening in this relationship involves considerable courage. The network CEO may become a target for each of the protagonists, who are more than ready to take on anyone who gets in their way even if it seems foolhardy to create conflict with the CEO. Similarly, one may attempt to use the CEO to gain some advantage. In this regard, successful intervention requires careful attention to interpersonal dynamics, which may come to include the CEO. The CEO can intervene by giving a direct order to end the combat and work together. This may work as both understand uses of power. Otherwise, care must be taken in helping these individuals put aside their interpersonal warfare by locating some benefit from the work that both will share in if they succeed in working together.

In the above example, the impasse and heated arguments eventually attracted the CEO's attention, and she decided to intervene by doing a little information gathering. She met with each of the two managers separately to learn more about each's perspective on the merger, progress or lack thereof, and the problems being encountered. No significant facilities, service, or operating problems seemed to exist. The problem appeared to rest in a power struggle between the two managers as to whose ideas were right and who would run the lab after the merger. The CEO decided that the GI lab manager would operate the new merged facility and that a steering committee composed of interested physicians and the surgery administrator would be formed to direct the lab's operations. The surgery administrator was thanked for his hard work over the years in building up the surgery lab and was asked to accept the decision and cooperate with the change. The CEO also indicated that once the merger was complete, the surgery service administrator would be asked to lead a team to start up in the network's new eating disorders program, which provided a reassuring note for the manager.

Arrogant-Vindictive versus Narcissist

The arrogant-vindictive executive is out to dominate the narcissist who prefers to be in the limelight to gain the attention and admiration of others, including the admiration of the arrogant-vindictive executive. The arrogant-vindictive executive, in contrast, is suspicious that others are out to get him or her and readily experiences the self-seeking and at times manipulative narcissist as threatening and, at the minimum, difficult to dominate. The arrogant-vindictive executive prefers winning, over being admired, while the narcissist prefers to be admired, over winning. However, the narcissist resists being dominated, which threatens his or her being seen as a person worthy of admiration, loyalty, and devotion. The resistance, however, may well fall short of a counterattack. The narcissist prefers to work behind the scenes to undermine opponents. This outcome is threatening to the arrogant-vindictive executive, who is invariably suspicious of those who do not come out in the open to take him or her on. The outcome of an ongoing relationship between these two executives is constant competition accompanied by open attacks and behind-the-scenes undermining.

The development of a new home healthcare product line may be seriously compromised by these two executives. The home healthcare arrogant-vindictive executive may become openly contemptuous of the narcissistic network executive, who is preoccupied with looking good and gaining attention. The arrogant-vindictive executive must try to dominate. Discussions about developing the product line may rapidly boil down to a battle of wills that everyone involved with the discussions knows about. Meeting participation and memos from the home healthcare executive often contain noticeably aggressive and contemptuous content that tends to polarize feelings even though some of the points being made are correct. The narcissist, however, is also intent on manipulating how others see his or her adversary and may be preoccupied with public posturing. He or she may also be particularly intent on trying to limit or get rid of his or her punishing colleague. This is accomplished by pressing the home healthcare executive to arrogant and contemptuous public behavior and working hard behind the scenes to cast this aggressive competitor in an unfavorable light, which might eventually compromise his or her career development if successful.

Intervention Strategy

This is once again a challenging intervention situation. Each adversary circles the other, carrying different instruments of self-fulfillment and destruction. What pleases one does not please the other. And, as noted above, this is another case where the intervening CEO is likely to be manipulated into supporting one over the other. The CEO may try to redirect their competitiveness toward him or her and enable them to work more effectively together so long as they are provided a clear direction and expectations for their work. This is a case where it is more difficult for a colleague or participant in the work to intervene. If the executives are not too anxious and mobilized and the situation has not existed for very long, a constant press of coaching may help to minimize the more destructive aspects of the relationship. The arrogant-vindictive executive can be encouraged to moderate his or her win-lose attitude in favor of win-win by collaborating. The narcissist can be encouraged to be less preoccupied with looking important and receiving admiration which, it can be pointed out, will come from a successful collaboration.

In the preceding example, the executives are locked in a hopeless self-defeating struggle that compromises the network's performance. The CEO intervened first by meeting individually with the highly mobilized competitors to look for some way to change their attitude and work to a win-win outcome. Each meeting required a similar firm approach. Each was confronted regarding documented behavior (often in the form of memos) that contained a competitive, win-lose nature. After gaining acceptance of this point of view (both may agree along some range but not fully embrace the notion that their approach to each other requires change,) the CEO unequivocally told each executive that cooperating with each other was expected. In extreme cases, a joint meeting may be held with the CEO to create a safer setting for each to commence constructive work with the other, with the CEO available to resolve major sticking points in the development of the new product line. If unsuccessful, the executive perceived to be the most resistant to changing his or her behavior or both may be reassigned, disciplined, sent for training, or terminated.

Arrogant-Vindictive versus Self-Effacing

This is an interpersonally workable match of psychological defensive tendencies. The arrogant-vindictive executive seeks to dominate and the self-effacing executive seeks to support others in return for being taken care of by them. Arrogant-vindictive executives hold contempt for those who are self-effacing (he or she abhors these tendencies in him- or herself). They also feel safe with this executive and occasionally become contemptuously abusive. The self-effacing executive is willing to accept some, if not considerable, abuse to maintain the relationship. This executive is willing to extend him- or herself to meet the needs of the other executive even if it is detrimental to him- or herself and his or her organization. The self-effacing executive will have a tendency to give up the shop in the face of stressful pressure and abuse from his or her arrogant-vindictive colleague.

A discussion as to which hospital will be selected for the development of a new cardiac catheterization lab will be dominated by the arrogant-vindictive executive from one of the hospitals, while the self-effacing representative from the second hospital is unassertive and may even be pushed into being supportive of the arrogant-vindictive executive's position. The result is publicly contentious behavior and memos on the part of the arrogant-vindictive executive that discourage colleagues from the other hospital, and others, from discussing and even thinking about asking a question or disagreeing. At the same time, the second executive is exceptionally passive, often trying to enlist her hospital CEO in the process.

Intervention Strategy

Interventions by the network CEO must focus on trying to maintain balance in the relationship. The arrogant-vindictive executive has to be discouraged from becoming too dominant and openly contemptuous, and the self-effacing executive must be encouraged to be more assertive and willing to represent his or her point of view. The CEO must not become entangled in the self-effacing executive's tendency to be admiring and dependent on anyone who seems willing to be a caretaker. This tendency, it must be noted, is exceptionally seductive in that it will make the CEO feel powerful, important, and needed by the executive. At the same time, caution must be exercised relative to the arrogant-vindictive executive who, if perceiving implied criticism and threat in the intervention, may be mobilized to perhaps unwisely challenge the network CEO.

In the above example, the CEO met with each executive separately to understand the point of view of each. Available documentation was reviewed with both. The CEO focused on the more blatantly aggressive win-lose behavior of the arrogant-vindictive executive by first identifying it and then indicating a change was necessary. Coaching suggested how to tone down the aggressive behavior as well as making it clear that being less aggressive was an expectation. Also discussed was that the goal of the work was a good, network-wide decision and that strongly advocating for one's hospital was not what was expected. The second self-effacing executive was encouraged to interact more assertively. It was pointed out that the executive from the other hospital had been asked to work in a more collaborative and less intimidating manner. Once again, it was pointed out that it was important that the decision optimize the network's performance.

Arrogant-Vindictive versus Resigned

This is a frustrating and unproductive pairing. The arrogant-vin-dictive executive wants to dominate; and the resigned executive, fears being dominated and constantly retreats from interaction with his or her colleague. The arrogant-vindictive executive is coercive, dominating, invasive, and threatening, which are all behaviors and personal attributes abhorred by the resigned ex-ecutive, who steadfastly avoids and withdraws from interactions that include them. As a result, the arrogant-vindictive executive becomes ever-more mobilized to overcome the retreat and re-mains in steadfast pursuit. The likely outcome is meetings that are not only difficult to arrange but that are combative and unproductive. The working relationship contains many impasses and administrative wastelands that are not really open for dis-cussion. Negotiations between an arrogant-vindictive network executive who is responsible for renovating a medical group's facility and a resigned executive of a medical group will be dominated by the arrogant-vindictive executive who will either get the medical group executive to agree to just about everything regarding the renovation or fail altogether to connect with the executive. Either outcome can ultimately cause negotiations to fail. The result may well be suboptimal renovation features that compromise the ability of the medical group's physicians to practice well or accept the change. Examining rooms may be too small for some portable equipment. Furniture may be dis-liked, or there may be insufficient work areas in the clinical space to complete medical records or read x-rays or for nursing staff to work.

Intervention Strategy

Successful interventions in this working relationship are difficult. The arrogant-vindictive executive is openly contemptuous of his or her resigned colleague, who is more than able to assert that the arrogant-vindictive executive is out of line. Changing this dynamic from an unproductive lose-lose to a more productive win-lose (the arrogant-vindictive executive has his or her way) to the most productive win-win (where the resigned executive is assertive and effectively represents his or her interests) requires providing the resigned executive training and coaching in how to be assertive as well as some supervised interactions to help each executive be more effective in working together. However, the resigned executive is likely to perceive a coercive influence in the CEO's intervention, and the arrogant-vindictive executive is likely to perceive a threat. The CEO will have to constantly monitor their working relationships, which is time-consuming and can be unrewarding. These executives may respond by further retreating to their defensive tendencies, which will make it just that much more difficult to get them to work together.

Arrogant-Vindictive versus Intentionalist

Arrogant-vindictive executives find their intentional colleagues hard to understand. The intentionalist seems unaccountably resistant to being dominated and to being drawn into combative win-lose dynamics—the familiar turf of the arrogant-vindictive executive. The arrogant-vindictive executive ultimately fears that he or she is being outmaneuvered by the intentionalist, who appears to be relatively calm and thoughtful, which, by comparison, may make the arrogant-vindictive executive look bad. The intentionalist is able to effectively deal with his or her arrogant-vindictive colleague by understanding the executive's underlying motivations and not reacting to them and his or her occasionally vindictive behavior unless clear harm is being done. The intentionalist defends him- or herself when appropriate. An intentionalist network executive who is trying to negotiate a preferred provider contract with a large employer will find the going tough when dealing with the arrogant-vindictive corporate executive who always wants more concessions. The executive may threaten to drop the negotiations, go to the network's CEO, or occasionally yell and slam doors. The intentional executive must be able to tolerate periodically demanding and even abusive behavior without taking personal offense even if the corporate executive personalizes his or her attacks. The intentional executive succeeds by trying to develop the relationship by making the corporate executive feel secure as well as paying close attention to his or her demands and trying to meet many of them in some way. At the same time, he or she also has firm limits as to how much abusive behavior is acceptable before contesting it (which builds reluctant respect on the part of the corporate executive) and is willing to patiently present and defend his or her point of view during the negotiations.

Intervention Strategy

Interventions by the network CEO may occasionally be needed as the intentionalist is not always able to limit the destructive aspects of an arrogant-vindictive colleague's behavior. The CEO may have to intervene in the negotiation to curb win-lose dynamics that the arrogant-vindictive executive brings to the negotiating table. The presence of the CEO may well flatter the corporate executive who prefers to deal with other powerful people, indirectly increasing his or her status by association. The CEO, however, may have to make it perfectly clear what the network's negotiating goals are in developing a preferred provider organization and for the executive's corporation and that if success is desired, the executive has to settle down and work on the task. Care, however, must be taken to avoid injuries to his or her excessive pride to avoid promoting more vindictive behavior.

Narcissist versus Narcissist

These executives find working together to be an interesting and rewarding experience. They enjoy swapping many expansive ideas, and will expend considerable time and energy discussing and developing grand schemes. However, the pairing can be unproductive in that they prefer ideas over action and do not like dealing with the details involved with implementation. Those responsible for operations find them unaccountably uninterested in dealing with the specifics of major operating problems. Rather, their response is to develop yet more ideas that promise to improve the situation. A narcissist network executive paired with a narcissistic hospital executive to develop a new ambulatory facility may well produce plans of a larger scope than initially anticipated, necessitating their reduction. These executives will also encounter difficulty in implementing the plan as unaddressed problems and details of implementation gradually pile up.

Intervention Strategy

The challenge of working with these executives is to gain the benefits of their expansive thinking while avoiding the pitfalls of their lack of attention to detail. These executives must be encouraged by the CEO to develop the interest and skills to deal with the managerial details of operations. Their work can also be facilitated by including others who have demonstrated skills in developing and implementing detailed plans. Their inclusion also promotes learning the needed skills to implement their ideas in the future.

In the above example, the CEO coached the two executives by critiquing their plans and requesting more information and specifics. The CEO provided helpful suggestions on the process of perfecting their plans, where to get information, where to seek help, and how to lay out their proposals. The executives were eager to please the CEO and worked hard to develop a more complete proposal for the new ambulatory facility. As the plans moved toward implementation, the CEO decided to create a task force that included the two executives as co-chairs and a number of additional staff who had considerable experience in operations of ambulatory facilities.

Narcissist versus Self-Effacing

These two executives create a strong pairing. The narcissist's need to feel admired and even loved are fulfilled by the self-effacing executive, who seeks to admire and serve someone who is willing to take charge. The narcissist is willing to take charge and leave the details for the self-effacing executive to handle. The self-effacing executive, in return for being taken care of, is more than willing to try to handle the details. Each benefits from the other's defensive tendencies. However, it is also likely that this pair will produce grand plans and ideas that are disconnected from reality and they can become defensive of each other, which can make them hard for others to deal with when they are together. A narcissistic hospital executive and a self-effacing ambulatory facility executive will develop major undertakings that are demanding to implement and maintain. The self-effacing executive is, in turn, expected to take care of the details of implementation and operations while his or her counterpart takes all the credit.

Intervention Strategy

Interventions may not be needed unless the self-effacing executive consistently fails to be assertive in representing his or her interests or underrepresents his or her organization or area or unless the narcissist comes to feel so expansive that he or she does not have to take into account his or her colleague's interests. A second possible imbalance may arise as a result of the narcissistic executive constantly producing a large number of visionary and complex schemes that the self-effacing executive dutifully tries to deal with. This results in the self-effacing executive being overwhelmed by the resulting work load. The executive is unwilling to confront the colleague about the problems his or her many ideas create.

In these cases, the network CEO must prioritize their work and insist it is on task and fulfills network goals. In particular, the narcissistic executive must be reminded that expansive plans are hard to implement and that if he or she is not going to get involved in their implementation, care must be taken to not overload those who assume responsibility for their implementation. In contrast, the self-effacing executive must be encouraged to provide feedback to his or her expansive colleague that grounds the dreams in the reality and limitations of the healthcare workplace.

Narcissist versus Resigned

These two executives find their working relationship unfulfilling. The resigned executive meets few of the narcissist's needs to be admired and does not manage the details of the work, but instead retreats both from the relationship and from responsibility for the work. The more the narcissist seeks the admiration of the resigned executive, the more his or her needs are rebuffed. This frustration leads to the constant pursuit of the resigned executive and perhaps to eventual abandonment of the relationship. In contrast, the resigned executive experiences the narcissist's many interpersonal needs to be a coercive influence that he or she is not about to become involved in meeting. This results in ever greater resistance to providing the narcissist with what he or she wants and in a willingness to avoid if not abandon the relationship. A narcissistic hospital CEO and a resigned healthcare system planner working together to develop a new product line will develop a frustrating and even bitter working relationship, which may compromise the project.

The CEO constantly generates new ideas, improvements, and changes to existing plans for the product line without much regard for the network planner's time or ideas. Efforts by the planner to fit the CEO's ideas to the network's strategic plan are often disregarded as are efforts to make the plans more realistic. Gradually the planner feels ignored and even set upon and gradually withdraws from the work and trying to work with the hospital CEO despite the fact that there is a firm time boundary for producing the plan. The CEO often speaks of the plan coming right along, while the planner says nothing in meetings where the plan is discussed.

Intervention Strategy

Interventions must focus on restoring a balanced interactive relationship. The network CEO may find it productive to schedule working sessions with the two executives and thereby overcome the resistance of each to working together. Colleagues and possibly consultants can coach these executives into working together by attending to some of the narcissist's needs for admiration by acknowledging that many of the ideas he or she has generated are good, while encouraging the resigned executive to participate in the work.

In the above example, the network CEO, during a meeting, provided the hospital CEO positive feedback on his ideas while also indicating that the details of the plan had to be worked out, which meant getting focused on the details. The planner, having heard this discussion with the CEO, was asked to produce the details of the plan by the expected date, directing particular attention at making sure the plans fit the network's overall strategy. Each executive left the meeting with a clear idea of what was expected.

Narcissist versus Intentionalist

This relationship is filled with tension. The narcissistic executive will not quite feel that the intentionalist executive is providing the unqualified admiration and attention that he or she deserves. The executive's efforts to gain attention and admiration are frequently ignored or rebuffed by the intentionalist, who prefers to deal with his or her narcissistic colleague based on how he or she is performing and not based on how he or she prefers to be seen and treated. The intentionalist also frustrates the narcissist's need to avoid dealing with details. The intentionalist avoids being drawn into meeting the narcissist's demanding needs unless the executive merits approval and admiration. The intentionalist is also aware of the narcissist's willingness to manipulate resources, decision making, information, and communication to reward him or her when he or she is suitably admiring.

A narcissistic network executive who is assigned the task of developing a new contract with the intentional CEO of a provider hospital finds the experience rewarding so long as the work progresses and the network executive receives approval from the network CEO. However, when difficulties are encountered, the narcissistic executive asserts that the intentional hospital CEO is hard to work with, as he or she never quite seems to appreciate the wisdom of the narcissist's grand ideas. The network executive eventually begins to manipulate reports of the CEO, taking credit for all of the work while at the same time criticizing the hospital's CEO. Eventually, the hospital CEO, takes exception with the network executive's representation and takes the issue up directly with the network CEO which is seen as a major threat to the network executive's reputation.

Intervention Strategy

This relationship works reasonably well, although the narcissist will invariably seek approval and admiration. The threat exists that the narcissist will come to feel overly frustrated and become organizationally destructive by being manipulative. The narcissist may also eventually reject the intentionalist and prefer to deal with someone else who promises to be approving and admiring and willing to take care of all of the details. These tendencies must be watched for and, should they occur, the narcissist must be encouraged to return to dealing directly with the intentionalist and avoid being manipulative.

In the above example, the network CEO reviewed the reports the network executive provided and compared them to the hospital CEO's explanation of the progress on the contract. The network CEO decided a meeting was necessary with her colleague to review the origins of some of the unresolved problems in the negotiation. The CEO appreciated the strong desire for her colleague to receive approval and carefully approached the discussion by first providing positive feedback on the negotiations and then providing some coaching on how to achieve closure on the remaining issues, which seemed to concern wrapping up many details and lose ends rather than anything substantive.

Self-Effacing versus Self-Effacing

Each of these executives depends upon the other to provide direction and to solve problems. Each, therefore, frustrates the dependency needs of the other. They will not enjoy working together, but they will not avoid it as each hopes that the other will eventually become the caretaker. Their collective lack of leadership and inability to produce good work leads them to seek the help of others, and consultants and other executives are a likely choice. A self-effacing executive of a diagnostic center will find it difficult to work with a self-effacing planner from the network when they are assigned the task of integrating the diagnostic center's patient registration and appointment scheduling systems with those of the network. Neither takes charge of the project; as a result, progress is slow and painstaking. Information system and planning specialists who work for the network and an external consultant are frequently called upon to locate the problems of the system integration, develop a plan of action, and then essentially carry out many steps in the plan. At times, these individuals are even asked to make major decisions, which in some cases they do.

Intervention Strategy

These two executives create a leadership and managerial vacuum that neither is willing to fill. If the void does not create operating problems, it may exist for considerable lengths of time. However, when the vacuum does create a problem, additional pressure results in these executives looking even more aggressively for the help of others. An intervention by the network CEO will inevitably fulfill their wish to be taken care of, as the CEO will end up being pulled into taking care of them and the situation if he or she is not careful or, at the minimum, will appear to fulfill their dependency needs by paying attention to them.

Avoiding promoting their dependency needs is important in an intervention. The CEO must steadfastly avoid solving the problems of the integration; however, he or she may play an active coaching or mentoring role. The two executives may, when coached, feel more self-confident and less self-effacing and as a result may be able to offer many of their own ideas as to how the project can be accomplished. The CEO can, through a series of meetings, coach these executives in their work, providing them a sense of safety while they experience themselves as effective, directive, and risk taking. The CEO essentially provides them a developmental opportunity.

Colleagues will, however, find these two executives frustrating to work with in that they invariably seem helpless and willing to let others take charge. This behavior draws colleagues into the role of doing their work and making decisions for them, which provides the desired caretaking behavior. Once again, avoiding the promotion of dependence is critical. Colleagues can also successfully coach their self-effacing colleagues into assuming risks, making decisions, and taking charge of their projects by helping them to organize their thinking and by reassuring them that they are on the right track.

Self-Effacing versus Resigned

The self-effacing executive seeks to be taken care of by others who take charge. His or her desire, however, is frustrated by the resigned executive who is simply unavailable to relate to and who does not want to take charge. The resigned executive finds the coercive expectations of the self-effacing executive to be nurtured, undesirable, and to be avoided. As a result, the resigned executive continually withdraws and avoids the self-effacing executive, who is constantly in pursuit. A self-effacing executive of a long-term care facility found developing additional financial and information processing resources from a resigned network executive difficult. The self-effacing executive, even though acting rather assertively, which was uncommon, found his resigned colleague remote and unavailable. As a result, the long-term care facility director readily felt rebuffed by his colleague and unable to engage her in a dialogue about the needed additional resources that would be critical if the facility was to meet network objectives set for the facility. Efforts to be assertive were met with avoidance and passive aggression from the network executive who made it clear that she would respond when she had time. Ultimately, facility renovations fell behind the scheduled expansion of the facilities services.

Intervention Strategy

These two executives created an unproductive pairing that required considerable intervention. Neither wanted to accept responsibility, and each found the other's actions frustrating and the person hard to work with. The interventions focused on minimizing each executive's tendencies to withdraw from responsibility. The intervention was well received by the self-effacing executive who saw the interventionist as someone who cared. In contrast, the resigned executive saw the interventionist as offering yet more coercive pressure which was to be avoided. As a result, intervention in this pairing was difficult, as was getting them to work together.

In the above example, the CEO decided to meet with both executives at the same time to review their progress. After receiving the progress report that documented that the changes in the facility were now months behind schedule, the CEO, while noting some disappointment in their progress, focused on having the two executives set new deadlines, which the CEO made clear were expected to be met. The CEO also responded to criticisms offered by each executive of the other. The self-effacing executive was asked to resume his efforts to work with the network executive while also being cautioned to avoid dependence. The network executive was asked to halt her avoidance of working with the facility executive and to accept the new deadlines even if she felt they were challenging or difficult to meet. The CEO also requested a progress report at the first of each month signed by both.

Self-Effacing versus Intentionalist

The self-effacing executive finds in the intentionalist someone who is willing to take charge and to provide nurturing, however, only up to a point. After that point, the intentional executive expects the self-effacing executive to manage situations and work without the desired immersion in a caretaking relationship. The intentional executive is aware of the self-effacing executive's control-oriented and flattering agenda of dependence and self-subordination, and avoids it. A self-effacing and usually unassertive home healthcare product line executive successfully negotiated the expansion of her product line with an intentional network executive who was asked to commit considerable additional network financial resources to purchase the needed equipment and vans.

Intervention Strategy

The intentionalist made this pairing work and provided a developmental opportunity for the self-effacing executive who was willing to accept responsibility for developing the needed resources under the guiding hand of the intentionalist. The intentionalist avoided being put into the position of carrying most of the responsibility, although his self-effacing colleague was more than happy to help out with the work associated with planning and financing the expansion effort. Had an intervention been necessary by the network CEO, he or she would have had to focus on aiding the self-effacing executive to become more independent, assertive, and willing to assume responsibility by providing some coaching on how to best accomplish the task at hand.

Resigned versus Resigned

These two executives want to be left alone and will, in turn, leave each other alone. As a result, their ability to collaborate and produce work is problematic, which will make everyone involved frustrated and anxious. These two defensive styles, however, might be compatible in a situation where hard-to-resolve interorganizational conflict exists and avoidance is preferred over resolution. A resigned hospital administrator and a resigned ambulatory facility administrator who have to work together to better integrate the inpatient and outpatient aspects of a service line will find each other willing to defend their own turf and avoid interacting to accomplish the work. As a result, minimal progress may be made in developing a comprehensive one-stop, cost-effective, patient-care-centered service. Each gradually becomes unwilling to give an inch or listen to what the other is saying. Each eventually becomes frustrated and angry and withdraws from interacting to get the work accomplished.

Intervention Strategy

Each of these executives wants to avoid the coercive influences of the other. A network CEO intervening in this relationship will find it hard to sustain contact with the two executives, who ultimately prefer to be left alone to do their own thing. Collaboration, therefore, comes only with the utmost effort. A general lack of success on their part may eventually result in either being directly ordered to work together or being dropped from leading the work.

Resigned versus Intentionalist

The resigned executive wants to be left alone and avoids coercive interactions. This executive continually withdraws from the intentional executive's efforts to interact; as a result, the intentional executive must try to work around the resigned executive's defensive tendencies. However, the resigned executive is also resistant to the intentionalist making any progress, as progress implies the coercive need for action on the part of the resigned executive. When the resigned executive of an old hospital owned by the network was approached by an intentional executive of the network with the notion of converting a number of his inpatient units to a respiratory care facility, he defended his turf and created a conflictual, defensive, and unpredictable situation, which only the patience and persistence of the intentional executive overcame. Many additional meetings and phone conversations were needed to assuage the hospital executive that the changes were not only necessary for the network to make, but that they would make his hospital more profitable and a noted regional center for respiratory care.

Intervention Strategy

Interventions by the network CEO must focus on encouraging the resigned executive to become a more responsible and an active participant. The CEO called a meeting with the resigned hospital executive to discuss progress or lack of progress on the conversion project. The meeting also presented her an opportunity to coach the executive in taking responsibility for the success of the change, and she eventually made it clear that the resigned executive was expected to assume responsibility for implementing the governing board's and her decision. A phone call to the intentionalist mentioned the meeting, and he was encouraged to persist in trying to get the work done.

Intentionalist versus Intentionalist

This is the ideal pairing of executives and is the type most commonly found. Each is self-reflective and able to work through anxiety-ridden aspects of work to find the best possible solutions. These executives are able to develop visions and ideas as well as work with the details of implementation. They are willing to accept change, take risks, and assume responsibility for their actions.

Conclusion

This chapter has taken an in-depth look at interpersonal behavior through the lens of the psychologically defensive tendencies described in Chapter 1. It must be appreciated that all of these psychologically defensive tendencies and their interactions change over time and even from moment to moment. An executive may at first hope to be admired for his or her grand ideas and failing that may experience an injury to his or her arrogant pride and strike out, seeking vindication for the injury. Win, lose, or draw, the executive may ultimately become hypercritical as his or her high performance standards go consistently unmet. Should none of these efforts reduce the executive's anxiety, he or she may withdraw. A defensive individual will rely on one strategy above others and use the other defensive strategies as needed to secure interpersonal control and relieve anxiety.

The chapter has in some ways underscored the obvious— that successfully working together under stressful workplace and competitive conditions can be difficult to accomplish and that when problems occur their origins can be difficult to understand.

However, all is not lost and indeed cannot be lost, as the work of integration must proceed.

Endnote

1. This chapter is based on the work of Michael A. Diamond and Seth Allcorn, "Psychological Dimensions of Role Use in Bureaucratic Organizations," *Organizational Dynamics* 14 (Summer 1985): 35–59; Michael A. Diamond and Seth Allcorn, "The Freudian Factor," *Personnel Journal* 69 (March 1990): 3, 52–65; and Karen Horney, *Neurosis and Human Growth* (New York: Norton, 1950).

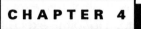

CHAPTER 4

UNDERSTANDING HOSPITALS AND MEDICAL GROUPS

Working effectively in the interpersonal world can be problematic when executives and employees become anxious and psychologically defensive. This chapter provides additional examples of psychologically defensive interpersonal interactions by examining hospitals and medical groups.[1] Keep in mind that psychologically defensive leadership styles are often present because of the stressful nature of management and leadership in hospitals and medical groups. However, it must also be appreciated that these defensive styles become exaggerated if the amount of stress is further increased, promoting even greater anxiety. A generally perfectionistic supervisor may become temporarily hypercritical if his or her management is criticized by a superior or if unexpected operating problems develop.

All of the interactions discussed in Chapter 3 will not be discussed here, just some of the more common ones found in hospitals and medical groups.

Working Together in Hospitals

The interpersonal arena in hospitals is filled with many professionals and tasks, creating extraordinary complexity. It is, therefore, important to have a conceptual scheme for understanding often unconsciously motivated interpersonal and role-to-role dynamics. This section explores the mastery-oriented, psychologically defensive responses to anxiety that result in a compelling need to take charge. The first response type mentioned in each section's subheadings is that of the executive, and the second is that of a subordinate. Hospital executives may also try to impose their psychologically defensive response to anxiety upward toward superiors and horizontally toward colleagues of approximately equal organizational rank. Intervention strategies are discussed from the point of view of a superior, usually a CEO, who intervenes in the dysfunctional work process that arises.

Perfectionist versus Perfectionist

A perfectionist hospital executive sets perfectionistic standards for his or her perfectionistic subordinates, which leads to a proliferation of alienating and unrealistic performance criteria. The result is that employees are constantly judged and criticized. Excessive attention is paid to unproductive and tedious detail which is grueling and encourages perfectionism from employees in order to avoid criticism. Some employees strive to receive approval by more perfectly meeting their superior's many expectations and standards. They may see the perfectionistic executive to be like themselves, striving for excellence and, therefore, someone to be admired. Others, however, may resist by imposing an alternate set of perfectionistic standards on their superior and his or her behavior and decisions, which invariably results in criticism. It is not important that the superior be aware of the standards and criticism in order for them to work to allay the anxiety of these employees.

This interpersonal dynamic is productive, but often wastes an employee's energy and time and frustrates superiors who try to control their employees. Accomplishing the task at hand becomes less important than perfecting every aspect of work on the task. Some parts of work need not be perfect in order to accomplish a task. An example is a clinical director of a large laboratory who is seldom pleased with the overall performance of the lab. Some employees become obsessed with achieving perfection and double and triple check test results, slowing down work and thereby adding new stress and criticism. Others may openly or privately criticize the director for being hypercritical and unrealistic about what can be accomplished given the staffing and equipment.

Intervention Strategy A senior executive who encounters these interpersonal dynamics finds some good news and some bad news. The good news is that everyone is striving to achieve a high level of performance. The bad news is that many employees are unhappy as the standards continue to be pushed ever higher by the lab director and may have, in fact, passed a point where they are achievable. The intervening hospital executive can begin by providing positive performance feedback to the director; he or she can review the high levels of consistently accurate and timely laboratory results the lab has been able to produce. However, the fact that some of the manager's performance standards are creating a problem with employee morale must also be addressed. Implications of criticism must be avoided, as the perfectionistic director will be sensitive to the lack of perceived perfection and control on his or her part. However, the reasonableness of the troublesome standards must be reviewed with an eye on compromise where appropriate. For example, a time standard that provides a result in 12 hours may be of no value for a physician who will not return to the hospital for another 24 hours to read the test results.

Perfectionist versus Arrogant-Vindictive

The perfectionist hospital executive frequently criticizes his or her arrogant-vindictive subordinates, thereby injuring their sensitive pride. In return, the subordinates counterattack and try to dominate or dispose of their superior. This interpersonal dynamic creates a combative working relationship. The executive tries to control his or her subordinates, who seem to be indifferent to what their superior thinks and feels. This executive's arrogant-vindictive subordinates hold contempt for their perfectionist superior who makes their work intolerable and who is seldom willing to fight back against their counterattacks other than by being more critical.

An example is a director of nursing who constantly criticizes her nurse managers, some of whom take strong offense to the criticism and the director. This subgroup of nurse managers are vocal about their problems with the director and have occasionally, as a group, complained to the hospital CEO. At the same time, the director is highly critical of this subgroup's attitude, behavior, and performance and has occasionally written disciplinary letters to some of them.

Intervention Strategy The CEO is confronted with a difficult mix of tendencies. These tendencies can create strong, polarized feelings that readily dominate discussions and efforts to create change. The CEO must coach the director of nursing into a less critical and punitive approach to dealing with his or her staff. The CEO must also make it clear to the subgroup of nurses that, if change is to occur, they must be a part of the process. A situation like this may be facilitated by external consultation and perhaps training such as team building. Executives and staff who possess these tendencies can accomplish good work when the relationships are in balance and the perfectionist superior monitors the much more aggressive and risk-taking work of these subordinates.

Perfectionist versus Narcissist

The perfectionist hospital executive seeks to impose restrictive, hard-to-meet standards on narcissistic subordinates who want to be admired and do not usually like detail. The promulgation of the detailed standards is accompanied by a tireless attention to them and frequent criticism does not make narcissistic subordinates feel good. Narcissistic subordinates may try to meet some of the standards to receive approval; however, they cannot consistently obtain it as the perfectionistic executive continues to hold out ever-higher standards. The best work is never quite good enough to receive unqualified approval. At the same time, the narcissist has little patience for details and prefers to work with the big picture, which infuriates the perfectionist.

These working relationships, however, can be productive. Narcissistic subordinates introduce creativity and risk taking that balance the perfectionist's preoccupation with control. On the other hand, work may not be accomplished if the perfectionist seeks ever greater control to combat anxiety, and narcissistic subordinates give up trying to receive approval and begin to defend against the executive's perfectionistic, critical, and micromanaging tendencies. Also to be considered is that the executive and subordinates may be weak on implementation where excessive attention to detail or lack of appreciation of detail become inhibitors. Similarly, implementation of change often requires forceful and effective leadership, which is something the narcissistic subordinates may avoid because of conflict and fear of losing their colleagues' admiration, and the perfectionist executive may compromise by being critical and unrewarding.

Interpersonal dynamics such as these might arise when an assistant vice president for operations sets unrealistically high performance standards for a cadre of senior level managers, some of whom feel there is a lack of overall planning and that there should be much more discussion of their ideas for improvements. They also feel inhibited by their superior's constant nitpicking of their proposals, which slows their progress to a crawl.

Intervention Strategy In the above example, the CEO will be obliged to intervene to review the performance standards with an eye to making them more realistic while avoiding making the vice president lose face or feel criticized or anxious. It is often difficult to adjust standards that are too high without appearing to promote mediocrity. One strategy is to set a series of standards that lead up to the very high standards. At the same time, the narcissistic subordinates need to be reminded that, while having lots of good ideas is important, it is equally important to produce quality work. This may be best accomplished by individual meetings with the CEO, who must sensitively but firmly make it clear to all of the executives that getting the work down is the primary task, not making it perfect or constantly changing it.

Arrogant-Vindictive versus Arrogant-Vindictive

This hospital executive may find him- or herself locked in a struggle for dominance and control of subordinates. They are suspicious of each other's motivations and may ultimately be out to eliminate each other. Their untrusting and highly competitive interactions reinforce these beliefs. Accomplishing work is subordinated to the struggle for dominance, which may result in high but perhaps uncoordinated productivity as everyone tries to outcompete and outproduce everyone else.

The working relationship is compromised by these arrogant-vindictive tendencies. The executive is confronted with subordinates who are unyielding in defending their point of view and willing to attack the executive's point of view. The executive is also equally unaccepting of the ideas of his or her subordinates. Little agreement occurs, which results in the executive ruthlessly dominating his or her subordinates, who fear this outcome and who are ready to actively or passively resist it.

These dynamics might arise around the hiring of a new CFO who immediately finds fault with how things are being done and orders major changes without discussing them with his or her immediate staff or with the those who manage departments. Some, if not many, of those challenged by the change are resentful of the implied criticism and offended by the unilateral tactics and begin to fight back in meetings and by complaining to the CEO. Interactions are continually contentious, as neither the CFO nor this group of executives and managers is willing to yield.

Intervention Strategy The CEO must change the punishing win-lose dynamics that have been created by the CFO's leadership style and the response of those executives and managers who prefer combative win-lose interactions. As is often the case, the CEO may only become involved after a history of dysfunctional interactions has been created and considerable animosity exists. It must be appreciated that the basic tendencies of these individuals militates against collaboration, as they often inject competition and win-lose dynamics into many of their interactions. In the example above, the CFO will be obliged to make it clear that collaboration is desired and that excessive interpersonal competition creates problems for all concerned. This may be accomplished by meeting with the CEO to discuss his or her leadership style and methods of introducing change. The CFO must be provided an opportunity to explain and perhaps ventilate about the development of the conflicted relationships that have arisen. Listening helps and must then be followed by coaching suggestions aimed at becoming more effective when acting as a change agent by, for example, including stakeholders in the decision making. Interventions with the other executives should be withheld in order to see if the CFO can succeed in making a leadership style change that provides the basis for spontaneously healing the conflicted relationships that have developed. If the situation is severe, outside intervention by consultants may be helpful as well as training in collaboration.

Arrogant-Vindictive versus Narcissist

The arrogant-vindictive hospital executive is suspicious of others and out to dominate narcissistic subordinates who like to receive attention and admiration. This executive prefers to win, while narcissistic subordinates resist being dominated because it threatens their self-image of being powerful and important. They resist by working behind the scenes to undermine the executive, which threatens the executive and reaffirms his or her suspicions that they are out to get him or her. The working relationship readily becomes one of constant competition and tension.

A take-charge autocratic hospital COO who is willing to do what is necessary to get the job done will find that many physicians with narcissistic qualities will resist his or her methods and leadership style. The COO's constant pursuit of his or her strategies through the use of power threatens this group of physicians, who also want to feel powerful and admired and who feel left out of decision making and participation in the operation of "their" hospital.

Intervention Strategy In the event these frictions cause dysfunctional behavior, the CEO must consider acting to encourage the COO to assume less of a win-lose leadership style, especially when dealing with the medical staff. This will involve finding suitable forums for including their participation in designing and implementing change. Open participation must be accompanied by a willingness to listen to what the participating physicians have to say and to compromise when appropriate. The COO, must be coached into a willingness to share decision making with the medical staff as well as perhaps with his or her immediate staff. Physicians must also be open to the prospect of change on the part of the COO and they must be encouraged to reflect upon their contribution to the problem.

Narcissist versus Narcissist

This hospital executive enjoys swapping ideas with narcissistic subordinates who also like to generate a lot of ideas and plans. These exchanges result in grandiose ideas and plans, but little work is accomplished and few actions are taken to make improvements. Operating problems may go unaddressed, as neither the executive nor the subordinates want to be confronted with the details of carrying out work or implementing the plans they generate.

For example, a COO and a number of his or her direct reports may spend hours in meetings discussing plans to implement total quality management and product lines, but may seldom reach decisions or set implementation in motion. Discussions lead to requests for research, to the hiring of consultants, and to continual announcements to other executives, managers, and staff, but not to action.

Intervention Strategy In this case, the CEO must intervene to remind the COO and the group that they must set firm time boundaries and then meet them. They can discuss their ideas as much as they have time to, but outcomes are expected. Simply asking for dates of implementation for agreed-to phases may be sufficient to keep work on a reasonable schedule without stripping the COO and his or her planning group of the pleasure of their many discussions, some of which produce positive benefits. A second aspect of an intervention may be to insure that the plans they generate are realistic, as this mix of narcissistic tendencies may generate grandiose plans. The plans may be overly ambitious, such as implementing a number of product lines at the same time or trying to incorporate a number of satellite clinics from the start. Plans may also be overly complex as many ideas become incorporated that do not exactly fit with other goals of the hospital. The CEO must steadfastly review the planning work as it proceeds in order to avoid wasting time and resources.

Working Together in Medical Groups

Medical groups are also filled with several types of psychologically defensive interpersonal behavior. Five of them are discussed below.

Perfectionist versus Narcissist

The perfectionist physician executive seeks to impose high and sometimes unattainable standards on work and others and is then willing to work tirelessly to achieve them. Others may experience these pursuits as overbearing, arbitrary, micromanaging, and coercive and may feel vulnerable to criticism. A physician executive who is responsible for a product line such as cardiology may set many standards for the performance of his or her colleagues and staff, who are then constantly monitored for compliance. Virtually every aspect of work is fair game for criticism. Attendance, speed of patient visits, patient waiting time, consumption of clinical resources, practice profiles, interactions with staff, billings, and patient satisfaction may all be carefully monitored. All of these aspects of practice are certainly important to monitor during these competitive and cost-conscious times. However, the perfectionist exceeds the reasonable by setting virtually unattainable standards, while becoming obsessed with collecting information. Colleagues and staff are confronted at every turn with evaluations and interventions, which they may experience as unfair and obtrusive.

Intervention Strategy The medical group's CEO and perhaps the medical group manager will usually learn about this type of behavior from complaints from colleagues and staff. Because the perfectionist often deals with written standards and data, other physicians and staff will be able to point to concrete examples of what they mean by excessive standards and interventions. Time must be taken to review the materials carefully. There are those cases where the standards are needed and reasonable and necessary; physicians and staff are only opposed to them because they mean more—but still reasonable— amounts of work. It is important to review the standards the physician executive has set and all other performance data that he or she has collected before reacting. This might be accomplished via a request for an orientation to the physician executive's area of responsibility. Standards that appear to be excessively high, standards that are constantly being raised so that no one is ever good enough, excessive reliance on rules and regulations, and the appearance of constant micromanagement are all indicators that the executive is coping with his or her anxiety about being a leader by enforcing perfectionism.

The intervention may be as simple as the CEO expressing approval of the executive's work and indicating that the work does not have to be approached with as much rigor as the physician executive is currently applying. There are, however, those who have a hard time overcoming their perfectionism because it makes them feel better about themselves as compared to others. Physician executives who have this tendency have to be coached and monitored. They can also benefit from leadership training and mentoring. Care must also be taken to avoid making these executives more anxious by implying criticism, which may be greeted with more perfectionism.

Arrogant-Vindictive versus Perfectionist

Some physicians can be overbearing and arrogant. When challenged, these physicians often think nothing of verbally attacking others, throwing objects, or kicking over waste cans. At the same time, they do not expect to be held accountable for their actions. A physician executive who possesses these tendencies will often be infuriated by the constant criticism and his or her implied inferiority relative to, for example, a perfectionist executive colleague in another specialty. Their interactions may often degenerate into win-lose dynamics. They just can't seem to work together for the betterment of the medical group. The head of a cardiovascular surgery team may constantly feel insulted and angered by the head of cardiology who constantly complains about the conduct and work of the surgeons. The surgeons, it is asserted, are unappreciative of the referrals they receive from the cardiologists and even demand more referrals. The cardiologist may also point out that some surgeons inappropriately intervene in the work of cardiologists who care for the cardiovascular surgery patients, which compromises their carefully calculated care programs.

Intervention Strategy These dynamics can often seem difficult to change because they are so ingrained. One of the keys is to intervene early before there are too many injuries on either side. Early intervention will make it clear that working together is important to their mutual success as well as to the medical group's success. In the event that considerable animosity has built up, interventions, while not ignoring this fact, must focus on change that will make the future better. Firm handling by the

111

CEO is essential, as may be follow-up sessions to discuss and monitor progress. Team-building training may be appropriate as well as work assignments with the CEO where these executives have to work together to solve mutual problems.

Arrogant-Vindictive versus Narcissist

The arrogant-vindictive physician executive sees him- or herself as better than others and is willing to attack others to make this clear. At the same time, narcissistic colleagues want to be liked and admired and to receive attention, which is enhanced by powerful roles and the propagation of grand ideas. An arrogant-vindictive physician executive who happens to supervise a narcissistic subordinate will often develop conflictual relationships with him or her. The arrogant-vindictive executive may not feel that he or she is likable and may resent his or her narcissistic colleague's efforts to be liked. At the same time, he or she is suspicious of the narcissist, who is willing to be manipulative and is unwilling to submit to the executive's authority.

These interactions may occur when an established, senior, arrogant, male surgeon and physician executive is confronted with a new female colleague who wants to be liked and admired by others. He seeks to dominate her, which she steadfastly resists. She provokes his suspicion by focusing on being liked by others. Her behavior threatens his role as an executive since he has certainly not gone out of his way to be liked by anyone and therefore feels vulnerable to being displaced. At the same time, her status as his victim creates favorable attention for her and some caretaking behavior on the part of others.

Intervention Strategy The CEO of the medical group is faced with difficult interpersonal dynamics that can produce a lot of dysfunction for the medical group and patient care if allowed to get out of hand. These two individuals operate in almost diametrically opposed ways, and each may well abhor the behavior of the other. Interventions can range from trying to avoid having them work together on committees and other situations where mutual respect and cooperation are prerequisites for success, to reassigning one of them to a different location. The middle ground involves trying to coach both of them into less defensive positions by having them work together in some type of structured setting, perhaps under the guidance of the CEO. During this process, the CEO would have an opportunity to learn more about the dysfunctional aspects of their working relationship and to intervene by drawing their attention to their competitive and manipulative behavior. Training, team-building exercises, opportunities to socialize, and outside consultation can also be of assistance.

Narcissist versus Narcissist

These individuals enjoy each other's company because they like to generate grand ideas and discuss the big picture. They are both, however, weak on implementation and prefer to avoid the messy details of acting on their ideas. It is often difficult to get closure with this pair, who prefer to continue to be creative even while implementation is underway, which may result in costly changes. Two of these physician executives in a committee will create a tendency to follow them into generating grandiose schemes, which are unrealistic and perhaps not part of the committee's task. The heads of oncology and nuclear medicine may constantly speak of developing a comprehensive cancer center when attention is really being focused on developing a new chemotherapy space.

Intervention Strategy Physician executives who posses narcissistic tendencies want to be liked and admired and like to talk about big plans. If they are confronted about their behavior by having its dysfunctional aspects pointed out, they usually modify their behavior as they do not wish to risk disapproval. In their minds, there is always a tomorrow to discuss their plans. They may also take their ideas outside of the group and try to convince others that they have merit, which may build a groundswell of support. To be avoided is threatening their preferred self-image of being liked, admired, and powerful.

Self-Effacing versus Perfectionist

The self-effacing physician executive prefers to be taken care of by others who are encouraged to take charge. While expressing an interest in what is going on and cheering colleagues and staff on, he or she is also unavailable to make major decisions and seems to avoid taking charge. In contrast, the perfectionist tries to stay in control by propagating many standards and holding people accountable. For example, a self-effacing physician executive will find a perfectionistic colleague is worth supporting in what, on the surface, appears to be the pursuit of excellence. The perfectionist is provided considerable latitude to pursue his or her agenda, which includes criticizing and possibly holding in contempt his or her self-effacing superior, who just does not take charge.

An example of this interaction is a physician executive who is assigned responsibility for developing a home healthcare program. He or she immediately recruits a take-charge physician from a similar program in a nearby city. Most staff are not hired until the new physician is on board, after which much progress occurs. Both physicians are pleased with the work; however, it becomes apparent that the new physician is the driving force in the program. This raises the question for the medical group's leadership as to whether to reassign their colleague, who was supposed to be in charge of the program, to a new task.

Intervention Strategy Interventions must focus on the overwhelming influence the perfectionist has on the work and the consistent willingness of the self-effacing executive to avoid giving direction and assuming responsibility. The self-effacing executive may be viewed as someone who is a good team builder because he or she promotes efforts by others to take charge. However, in the long run, this executive compromises departments and programs he or she is in charge of by not providing strong direction. It is equally likely that some of those who are providing the direction will eventually resent the executive and seek to replace him or her. At the same time, a colleague who is a perfectionist may eventually not have his or her perfectionism reigned in when it becomes dysfunctional. Therefore, initially the self-effacing executive may be left in place to build a team, but colleagues such as perfectionists may require interventions by the CEO if their tendencies become overdetermined and dysfunctional. In the long-run, the self-effacing executive may be reassigned to a new project where he or she will once again try to recruit take-charge colleagues.

Conclusion

This chapter examined some of the complexities of working together in hospitals and medical groups that have their origins in psychologically defensive responses to the experience of excessive anxiety. The examples and problems discussed and the suggested intervention strategies provided offer a new and more systematic way to understand and cope with these types of dysfunctional behaviors that compromise being able to work together effectively in the ever-more stressful healthcare delivery workplace. The suggested intervention strategies offer new insights into how to successfully overcome psychologically defensive workplace dysfunctions once they develop and begin to adversely affect collaboration and work.

Endnote

1. This chapter is based on the work of Michael A. Diamond and Seth Allcorn, "Psychological Dimensions of Role Use in Bureaucratic Organizations," *Organizational Dynamics* 14 (Summer 1985): 35–59; Michael A. Diamond and Seth Allcorn, "The Freudian Factor," *Personnel Journal* 69 (March 1990): 3, 52–65; and Karen Horney, *Neurosis and Human Growth* (New York: Norton, 1950).

CHAPTER 5

GROUP AND ORGANIZATIONAL CULTURE

Developing and managing a large, complex, fully-integrated healthcare delivery network is stressful and challenging. The problems that size and complexity present are often further aggravated by the presence of many different group and organizational subcultures that contain within them psychologically defensive and potentially dysfunctional aspects aimed at controlling employee anxieties about themselves, others, their jobs, and the organization. Multiple hospitals, medical groups, ambulatory facilities, long-term care facilities, and home healthcare organizations each have an organizational culture that contains some dysfunctional elements. Some groups of employees, such as physicians, nurses, and therapists, have values and methods that create a culture uniquely suited to their interests and that helps them to defend against their anxieties. Other functional groupings of employees—such as those who manage product lines, appointments and scheduling, reception, medical records, billing, relationships with third parties and nonsystem hospitals and clinics, vendors, planning, finance, information systems, benefits, and facilities—also develop group cultures that contain psychologically defensive elements. Understanding the psychological side of how the network culture and its many subcultures function is important if cost-effective quality is to be achieved.

Definitions

In order to be effective at leading and managing a network, a hospital or medical group must first have a clear idea of what the psychological side of group and organizational culture is and how it is created. Group and organizational cultures are unconsciously invented, discovered, or developed patterns of basic assumptions that limit member anxiety. In effect, they become an important externalized social defense mechanism that controls experience and limits anxiety. These basic assumptions permit their members to cope with anxiety-provoking problems of adapting to the external operating environment while also permitting sufficient internal integration to make collaborative work feasible.[1] What works is then taught to new members as the correct way to perceive, think, feel, and act at work.

This description of group and organizational culture contains several important elements. First, it includes a pattern of unconscious basic assumptions about human nature that are not particularly open to inspection or questioning and must often be deduced. Despite their lack of visibility, these unacknowledged basic assumptions shape perception, thinking, and feeling. Group and organization members come to understand, outside of conscious awareness, what basic assumptions govern working relationships, including how they understand human nature; what motivates people at work; and the nature of the relationship of the network, hospital, medical group, or other subgroup to its operating environment. These assumptions minimize conflict and limit anxiety. The substance and philosophical nature of these basic assumptions are discussed in Chapters 7 and 8. The focus in this chapter and the next is their unconscious origins and the types of group and organizational cultures they may create.

Organizational culture arises from the unconscious assumptions shared by the healthcare and physician executives who develop and operate integrated networks and those who lead their subdivisions (which have their own subcultures). As noted in Chapters 3 and 4, assumptions, philosophies, and world views held by organization members are heavily influenced by prior life experience and unconscious conflict and at times by psychologically defensive motivations that distort thinking and feeling. These conflicts and resulting distortions ultimately influence the assumptions held about oneself, others, the organization, and the world—assumptions that also unconsciously influence what we sense, think, feel, and relate to others. These shared systems of unconscious thinking and feeling form much of the basis for the psychologically defensive types of group cultures described in this chapter and the next.

These shared systems of unconscious thoughts and feelings are introduced into the workplace through the personalities and psychologically defensive tendencies of healthcare and physician executives and gradually become shared by others because these executives influence everyone's thoughts and feelings. The result of this unconscious interpersonal contagion is a set of mutually agreeable thoughts, feelings, and actions that regulate personal and interpersonal anxiety. Those working with the executive begin to share many of the same thoughts and feelings without being aware of it. Those who do not like the process and the content of the thoughts and feelings often leave or drop out of active participation. As a result, these patterns of thinking, feeling, and experience gradually become the unquestioned rituals, protocols, and myths and fantasies that shape perception, experience, thoughts, feelings, and actions. They, in effect, are the unconscious foundation upon which network cultures are built.

There is an endless array of examples of how the unconscious nature of organizations develops and changes. The following example begins with the hiring of a new network executive responsible for developing the seamless integration of networked hospital and medical group medical records and databases.

Sarah is the only child of two highly successful executives who were too busy to be with her very often as she grew up. When they were with her, they dominated her life. Sarah vacillated between feeling unworthy of their attention and abandoned, or imperfect and requiring constant direction and supervision. As Sarah grew up, she became preoccupied with controlling how close people were to her (interpersonal distance), and as an adult she feels very anxious when superiors, subordinates, and colleagues seem too distant or take too much interest in her work and decisions.

When Sarah began her network position, she immediately and unwittingly introduced her need to maintain the correct interpersonal distance into her work and working relationships. Those around her quickly learned that she needed to feel worthy and admired (the narcissistic response to anxiety) but also that she took offense if they took too much interest in her (the resigned response).

Gradually, her staff became preoccupied with meeting her need to maintain the proper interpersonal distance and with making her feel admired and valued. Work processes and reports were modified to fulfill these needs. Bad news was seldom communicated to her, and her occasional poor decisions were seldom vigorously questioned to avoid upsetting her. Her staff eventually found themselves trying to take care of her and each other. They absorbed most of the problems, to which Sarah's marginal decisions often contributed. As a result, her staff gradually became risk averse and unwilling to confront problems and tough issues. They implicitly knew that if they could not solve the problem, Sarah would become anxious and blame it on them. Major operating and integration issues were consistently avoided, which gradually but continuously compromised their efforts to develop a seamless network of participating hospital and medical group information systems.

Everyone involved felt unsupported and locked into double binds because Sarah was unwilling to intervene to make unpopular decisions out of fear of losing the admiration of others. These many unconscious interpersonal and group dynamics were shared by most of her staff as well as those managing the information systems of the network's hospitals. Sarah's department was known as overly concerned with the quality of interpersonal and group relationships to the detriment of making the tough and possibly unpopular decisions that occasionally have to be made to achieve information system conformity. These individual, inter-personal, and group dynamics determined how Sarah's em-ployee's saw themselves and their work world, what work is really about, and how people should relate to each other. The uncon-scious elements became the brick and mortar of an organizational subculture.

Organizational culture is also created from learning what works. It evolves from experience, which permits change and adaptation relative to the open system in which it exists. If a behavior or way of thinking or feeling does not work, it is not adopted; and if it eventually fails to work, it is abandoned, although rigid hierarchical and bureaucratic process and isolated autocratic leaders may block or subvert change even when there is clear evidence of failure. As a result, once an element of culture is established as dependable, it may not be promptly changed or deleted even if it is known to be dysfunctional. The irrational psychologically defensive side of organizational life often perpetu-ates unacknowledged but familiar assumptions, processes, and relationships that may have grown inconsistent with the changing operating environment because everyone is afraid of losing what is familiar.

A CEO might decide to tap the creative energy of the hospi-tal's staff and ask them to also provide vision and direction. However, if their ideas always have to be brought to the CEO for review, assessment, and approval, nothing much has really changed, and the hospital remains strangled by its "great man" culture. The cult of the CEO still dominates the hospital and the idea of allowing more participation on the part of the hospital's staff does not, in effect, exist. The hospital's culture has not changed and has, in fact, built in a dysfunctional double standard that its members learn exists.

The questions raised by this discussion of the psychological side of organizational culture are What are the governing assumptions of the culture? Are they internally consistent? How do they make the network, hospital medical group, and their constituent subcultures different from those of other organizations? These are important questions to reflect upon as you read this chapter and Chapter 6.

The Psychological Foundation of Group and Organizational Culture

The premise of this chapter is that employees create a culture to reduce the anxiety that arises when they are confronted with complexity and uncertainty. Being anxious is natural, given the complex internal and external operating environments of integrated healthcare delivery organizations, hospitals, and medical groups. Anxiety must be reduced to tolerable levels to avoid becoming emotionally overwhelmed and unable to act. Group and organizational culture helps to make work life more predictable by shaping thinking and feeling and filtering out extraneous variables. In particular, culture reduces anxiety about what is going on inside of the network, hospital, or medical group and what is going on outside during these turbulent times.

Limiting "Inside" Anxiety

Inside anxiety is that aspect of the healthcare workplace that makes organization members anxious but that is for the most part within their control. Networks, hospitals, and medical groups are composed of people who relate to each other through roles that create predictability and trust and that minimize anxiety and uncertainty. Working inside of a network, hospital, or medical group can also be threatening and anxiety ridden if work gets out of control. Getting everyone on track and working together creates internal integration that minimizes anxiety and psychological defensiveness. Factors that limit inside anxiety are (1) a common language and ways of thinking and understanding events; (2) clear group boundaries and roles, including how one becomes a member and how others are excluded; (3) an understanding of how power and status are acquired; (4) intimacy, friendship, and love; (5) a system of rewards and punishments; and (6) an ideology or "religion." These aspects of organizational life bind people together, improve predictability, and provide some measure of interpersonal control.

Healthcare and physician executives, managers, and employees deal with these aspects of organizational life daily but are not usually aware of them in these terms. Organization members need a common understanding of what is going on, and what is being said and done, and they must be able to arrive at some level of consensus as to what needs to be done, how, and by whom. Achieving this understanding is aided by their sharing a common knowledge and language.

Members of networks, hospitals, and medical groups must also understand where their respective organizations and subgroups end and where they, others, and the operating environment begin. Confused and internally inconsistent statements about what the organization is and how it works create conflict that is difficult to resolve and that drains valuable creative and productive energy. Clear statements about what the network, hospital, and medical group consists of, its values, and how success is determined, as well as clear organizational boundaries and criteria for membership, increase predictability and minimize ambiguity, risk, and anxiety. Executives, managers, and employees must also know where they fit into the scheme of things to enable them to experience meaningful membership and to be able to effectively contribute. This is, of course, made all the more difficult by the advent of networks that assemble a hard-to-understand and ever-changing array of hospitals, medical groups, third parties, and other healthcare related enterprises.

Network, hospital, and medical group members must also understand how power and authority are allocated and used.

Power and authority often threaten organizational attributes that are important to conserve and use wisely. Employees need to feel assured they will not become the focal point for the aggressive or destructive use of power and authority. Organization members need to feel they have control over their work in order to avoid feeling dependent, infantalized, and ineffective.

Network, hospital, and medical group members also want to feel valued and even loved, especially during downsizing and reengineering. The desire to be friendly and supportive draws people together while suspicion, anger, shame, and doubt drive them apart. Healthcare and physician executives must encourage teamwork. They must make it clear that they respect the thoughts, feelings, and contributions of those who work for them or, better, with them. They must make it safe to speak up, try new things, and assume risks.

Rewards and punishments must be understood and wielded in a fair and predictable manner to make staff feel safe and wanted in the workplace; they must also support goals and discourage actions, thoughts, and feelings that are inconsistent with achieving them. Finally, networks, hospitals, and medical groups are filled with stories and myths that elaborate the ideal image of the organization, its employees, and their work. Networks, hospitals, and medical groups have their heroes, who have accomplished great feats in the toughest of circumstances. Organization members have suffered through great organizational victories as well as tragedies and defeats. These stories and myths contain a great deal of meaning that helps to direct thinking, feeling, and action toward the organizational ideal and what is valued by top management and the employees of the network, hospital, or medical group. They become part of the history and fabric of the organization that every employee learns about and by doing so learns how to adjust thinking, feeling, and actions to those that are valued.

All of these aspects of networks, hospitals, and medical groups make participating in them less anxiety ridden and, therefore, less likely to provoke psychological defensiveness. Hospital and physician executives must promote good feelings about self, others, work, and the organizations. This desirable state is, however, hard to achieve; and for some networks, hospitals, and medical groups, the reality of the "inside" falls far short of these ideals. The results are commonplace. Physicians may constantly contest the control exerted by healthcare executives over allocation of resources. Autocratic, top-down decision making that violates organizational boundaries and personal authority and disempowers virtually everyone may abound. Some employees are rewarded for the unquestioning compliance; whereas, others who question decisions and authority are singled out for abuse. Networks, hospitals, and medical groups filled with internal dynamics such as these increase anxiety and psychological defensiveness, compromising their ability to achieve success.

Limiting "Outside" Anxiety

Outside anxiety is that part of the healthcare workplace that is external to the network, hospital, or medical group and, therefore, beyond its immediate control. Integrated healthcare organizations must, in addition to having an internal order that limits anxiety, chaos, psychological defensiveness, and self-defeating behavior, be able to cope with an operating environment that is filled with competitors, informed healthcare consumers, government, employers, and managed care organizations, all of which introduce a myriad of conflicting pressures that are difficult to manage. Organizational elements that permit the members of networks, hospitals, and medical groups to cope with anxiety arising from conflicting external pressures must also be successfully dealt with in order to assure survival. These elements include (1) an organizational mission and strategy, (2) goals that fulfill the mission, (3) organizational resources to accomplish the goals, (4) a way to measure success, and (5) a process of correction when measurement indicates work is not fulfilling goals. These common elements of management provide networks, hospitals, and medical groups with a unified purpose and direction that, if successfully carried out, permit survival and even success in the external world. Executives, managers, and employees deal with these organizational elements daily as they dictate what everyone is supposed to be doing and toward what planned end. They are also likely to contain many of the irrational elements of organizational life by limiting anxiety about what is happening to the network, hospital, or medical group and how it will respond.

The leaders of fully integrated healthcare organizations must envision and communicate a mission for their organization. A universally understood mission creates a shared understanding that influences the thinking, feeling, and actions of employees. Likewise, strategies that operationalize the mission further instruct thinking and feeling and guide managers, administrators, and workers in their actions. The mission and strategy are further operationalized in the form of internally consistent goals and congruent objectives. This "rational" process of boiling everything down to the essentials, however, often begins to break down as the willful and sometimes irrational behavior of organization members begins to create "off-task" political and power-oriented outcomes. A physician executive who continues to oppose a decision to merge her program with another department may either undermine the decision or her credibility. At the same time, she compromises the well-being of the hospital and network to effectively compete.

Even more individualized and, therefore, open to manipulation are the means of getting the work done to meet the objectives aimed at goal achievement. Means, while including resources, process, and methods, really begin and end with the overwhelming influence of the wielding of interpersonal power. People who feel they have to be in control to feel good about themselves can be depended upon to strive for power, which they then unconsciously seek to wield to meet their own needs. In the process network, hospital, or medical group resources may be used to gain and conserve power, and manipulated to acquire attention, admiration, and loyalty by essentially buying people off. Network planning may be subtly manipulated to reward a hospital CEO who is a close friend of the network CEO to the disadvantage of other network hospitals. Once again, the network's competitiveness may be diminished relative to its task environment.

Another aspect of management is that the results of work must be monitored and those responsible for the work should be held accountable, which may lead to fears of corrective action. These two steps, monitoring and corrective action, are often unconsciously associated with the experience of being held accountable by a parent. Being held accountable can carry with it feelings of being powerless, dependent, and punishable for not being good enough. Accountability, performance evaluation, and rewards and discipline are filled with negative feelings associated with guilt, shame, power, and dependency and are, as a result, often avoided by healthcare and physician executives or acted upon with ruthless indifference, either of which defends them from the experience of taking the action.

There is a circularity to these outside-oriented processes that constitutes a feedback loop. Organizational survival depends on a suitable mission and accompanying goals and objectives that are internalized by employees to guide them in their work. This awareness leads us to consider how the underlying fabric of integrated healthcare delivery organizations—their culture—contribute to operationalizing the mission. I now turn to the discussion of group and organizational culture.

Psychologically Defensive and Nondefensive Group and Organizational Cultures

Four types of group and organizational cultures are described below. Each culture has unique characteristics. Three of the cultures have psychologically defensive dysfunctional aspects to them that, while promising to control the anxieties of their members, ultimately make group life more, rather than less, stressful. The fourth nondefensive culture is provided to explain what a relatively nondefensive group or organizational culture is like.

The four catagories of group cultures apply equally well to the overall network as to hospitals, medical groups, ambulatory facilities, long-term care facilities, and home healthcare organizations. It is also important to appreciate that these subgroups of the network will be dominated by the integrated network's dynamics. What is going on in the system can be expected to involve everyone. Another important aspect of organizational and group cultures is that they are all dynamic, changing as members of the organization create new ways of dealing with the pressures of the healthcare workplace. A culture can change into another culture as member needs for security and self-esteem are frustrated by group processes or by internal or external forces. Change in the culture is inevitable over time.

In sum, the four types of organizational and group cultures provide insight into the true complexity that exists within groups and organizations and among organizations and groups. Intra-group and intergroup dynamics and the inevitability of change also serve to confound an overly simplistic understanding of group and organizational culture and dynamics. Each culture evolves from learning what works to relieve member anxiety in much the same way as individuals learn what psychological defenses allay anxiety. Each culture also implicitly answers the philosophical questions of what the group is; how it works; and how members are to think, feel, and act (discussed in Chapters 7 and 8).

Homogenized Group and Organizational Culture

This culture is familiar to medical groups and academic health sciences centers but less familiar to hospitals and networks. The culture arises from desires for autonomy and independence. Members protect themselves from each other by steadfastly maintaining their personal autonomy. Everyone is equal (a colleague); no one is better or more powerful. This culture is often symbolized by everyone sitting in a large circle, with the appearance of equality.

This culture, while clearly embedded within an identifiable group or organization, acts more like a crowd. The pursuit of autonomy creates a group that appears to lack, and may indeed lack, a clear purpose and effective leadership. Efforts to lead, either by the designated leader or by others, are not heeded. Homogenized group dynamics eventually discourage anyone from trying to lead the group or organization. These dynamics are epitomized by a medical group of 60 members where all of the members must approve a proposal before it is adopted.

When put under stress, however, homogenized group members readily feel the lack of connectedness to each other. They cut themselves off from each other to maintain their independence just when they could benefit from dealing with the anxiety-promoting problem together. Some employees will feel that they are neither in nor out of the group, which causes confusion and distress. They are there but do not feel apart of the group or what is going on. They feel that they can neither engage in the group nor separate from it. Inside anxiety abounds.

Anxiety is further enhanced by the group eventually losing touch with its purpose and its operating environment. It may act as though it has entered into a timeless, unchanging state, where nothing needs to be accomplished despite considerable evidence to the contrary. Reality testing is compromised as each member pursues his or her highest priority: maintaining personal autonomy and interpersonal safety. Outside anxiety, therefore, may also abound.

Gradually, group members come to feel angry with the group while also fearing what the group may do to them. The lack of connectedness and voluntary subordination, causes the group difficulty with accomplishing work on its tasks. Under these circumstances, withdrawing physically and psychologically becomes the safest thing to do (the resigned response). Individual members may also seek support and safety by pairing with other colleagues or by joining small subgroups of three or four individuals to create some sense of security (the self-effacing response).

If the group's members feel sufficiently threatened, there may be a change to one of the other types of group cultures if suitable leadership emerges and there are enough group members who are in enough pain to follow the leader in making the change.

The Case of Too Many Bulls in the Pasture Hospitals are run by executives who are used to making decisions. At the same time, physicians are used to running their own practice and are also interested in being left alone to practice medicine. The Greener Pastures Clinic (GPC) is a 40-physician multispecialty group with a number of strategically located clinics that are a natural fit to the territory of the Metropolis Health Care System (MHCS). The CEOs of both organizations are receptive to exploring the development of an integrated working relationship and appointed a half dozen senior level administrators to open discussions. Bob Willy, the executive vice president for MHCS System Development, it was agreed, would chair the working group. Dr. Brown was designated to lead GPC in its negotiations, as he was responsible for practice development.

The first meeting of the group, however, was not well attended by GPC personnel. One administrator and one physician showed up. It was explained that Dr. Brown and the other two physicians had emergencies they had to deal with. Bob Willy, thinking quickly to salvage the situation, used the meeting as an opportunity for them to get to know each other and to review the group's purpose. Little else was accomplished.

The second meeting two weeks later was attended by everyone. During the intervening two weeks, the idea of merging with MHCS had been exhaustively discussed among many of GPC's physicians. A number of polarizing points of view and problems had emerged from the discussions. Within 10 minutes of the start of the second meeting, chaos broke out. There were a number of one-on-one discussions taking place among the physician's and several MHCS executives. Efforts by Bob Willy and occasionally others to intervene had little effect on the willingness of group members to work as a group. They continued to intermittently argue their points of view with each other. Several physicians even challenged the appropriateness of Bob's role as chair. The meeting ended on time; however, a number of physicians continued their discussions in the hall after the meeting.

The third meeting started with Bob Willy trying to capture all the different points of view. However, within minutes arguments broke out as to whether this or that point was correct or should be included. A particularly divisive element implied in some of the discussions was a proposal that had just been received from a second system eager to merge with GPC. Many in the physician group believed that the new offer should be considered at the same time.

Every time the work group met, chaos erupted. Clearly, there was to be no meeting of minds. There was little agreement on the problems much less progress toward exploring the implications of the integration. Weeks passed without progress. Some analyses were developed, but they were disregarded.

The group was given an additional month to develop a recommendation but with predictable results. Interventions by MHCS's CEO also proved ineffective. It was ultimately concluded that the work group was not going to be able to reach any kind of consensus, and the integration effort was put on hold.

Case Analysis This is a good example of the chaos that can develop in homogenized groups. Many of the executives had their own points of view that could not be reconciled. Strong personalities discouraged collaboration and compromise. The case illustrates how autonomy issues can dominate a group and its work.

Intervention Strategy An outcome such as this is not uncommon. Inside and outside anxiety flooded the discussions. Work inside the task group was uncooperative and filled with unresolvable tension and conflict fed by outside anxiety involving the

131

loss of GPS's identity and mission should integration occur. Putting the discussions on hold will permit a cooling-off period in which the CEOs of GPC and MHCS will have an opportunity to explore and understand what happened to the discussions with their staff and to share their findings with each other. At this point, the route to successful integration is for the CEOs to work with their staffs to develop, as near as possible, concise criteria for integration and to then work with their colleagues to gain acceptance of the proposal. This will be facilitated within GPC by the presentation of information about changes in the market-place and the need for integration to insure long-term survival. Outside anxiety will promote greater group cohesion among the physicians of GPC. This strategy is essentially followed by Dr. Jones when the case is resumed in the next section.

Institutionalized Group and Organizational Culture

A homogenized group may, in an effort to get something done, follow the actions of its formal leader or an informal leader who promises to create a more structured approach. This approach promises to defend its members from group membership anxiety by creating rules, regulations, and formal roles that control all interactions. Everyone knows what he or she is to do, what others are to do, and the procedures by which work is to be accomplished. A hierarchical structure is developed where even the leader is not threatening, as he or she has to follow the rules of leadership agreed to by the group. The leader's role is, in effect, circumscribed and carefully and completely controlled. The ultimate goal of the institutionalized group is to control what its members think, feel, and do, including the leader. Rigidly "adhered" to protocol, paperwork (forms and formats), rules, and behavioral patterns offer everyone interpersonal safety and per-mit some work to be accomplished.

Institutionalized groups accomplish work but often at the cost of creativity, flexibility, and the ability to learn from experience. Big institutions are notorious for having difficulty adjusting to new circumstances. Members are expected to suppress their desires for autonomy; however, self-interest still continuously emerges in the form of organizational politics, self-protection, special interest groups, and power plays that disrupt carefully developed and controlled work plans and processes. This outcome, when combined with a lack of flexibility and poor learning, often ends up threatening the group's ability to accomplish its task. The group may, at this point, reinforce its institutionalized behavior with rules and process, or it might possibly evolve to another type of group if a leader is present to lead group members in change.

The Case of Doing It by the Book Institutionalized work groups are common in hospitals. Hospitals rely on institutionalized methods to coordinate the interactions of their many professions and services. At the same time, caregivers abhor the accompanying restrictive rules and paperwork that do not always yield the expected outcomes. In contrast, medical groups may have few business and work processes that can be consistently labeled institutional. Physicians do not like to have their practice of medicine controlled and, as noted, they disdain the burgeoning amount of paperwork. A large integrated healthcare delivery system faces the same problems that hospitals have in coordinating the actions of their many member organizations, some of whom are opposed to institutionalized processes.

GPC's inability to get its act sufficiently together to have a meaningful discussion with MHCS concerned Dr. Jones, CEO of GPC, who realized that the subspecialists and other departments of GPC were inevitably going to defend their turf. Ritualized combat between the generalists, subspecialties, and service departments abounded, and inside group anxieties were acted out in the meetings with MHCS. Dr. Jones appreciated Dr. Brown's valiant efforts to lead the negotiations; however, it was clear that Dr. Brown did not possess the force of personality needed to lead a consensus-building process within GPC.

Dr. Jones fully understood the need for GPC to join an integrated network to enhance its long-term survivability, and he decided to try to work out a decision through the clinic's well-established management structure. The proposal, which was by now common knowledge within the group, was presented for discussion at the next department heads' meeting. Dr. Jones requested a written assessment from each department head. Subsequent discussions at weekly meetings eventually led to a better understanding of why joining an integrated system was important, why MHCS's proposal was the best one on the table, and how integration was likely to affect the group. However, as the exciting new idea began to take form, many of those participating began to see implications for themselves and their departments. Joining MHCS would mean substantial changes for GPC and its many operations. After this point, meetings where the proposal was discussed became immersed in discussions of how integration would change and adversely affect current operations. Many of the physicians, managers, and employees were anxious and defensive about losing familiar and secure routines and working relationships. A small number of department heads were also becoming frustrated by what was becoming a justification of the status quo. Arguments for integration and change were increasingly greeted by the refrain, "Why do we need to change? We have always been successful."

It was about this time that Dr. Jones understood that the group was beginning to foreclose on its options by reinforcing its hard-won institutionalized processes. However, much work had been accomplished by evaluating the new opportunity. It was clear that integrating was necessary if GPC was to maintain marketplace viability in the future. A substantial threat existed that everyone was beginning to grudgingly admit to. It was also clear to Dr. Jones that moving forward from this point would require a leader who possessed a forceful personality, someone who could overcome the growing resistance to change. Dr. Jones selected Dr. Fellow to lead the group in the final negotiations with MHCS and eventual integration. Dr. Fellow had risen to prominence during department head meetings as a strong and effective advocate for integration. She had also developed a loyal following among those who were supporters of the idea.

Case Analysis The case illustrates that conventional organizational precepts that provide structure and routinize behavior can produce a viable organization. Everyone works together under the direction of a well-understood and accepted leader. However, discussion of change is threatening to the established order and promotes inside anxiety. The greater the inevitability of change and accompanying anxiety, the greater the psychological defensiveness and resistance.

Intervention Strategy The use of familiar roles, including that of Dr. Jones, and organizational process within GPC calmed internal anxiety sufficiently to permit GPC's members to focus on the external threat and anxiety and their need to change in order to integrate with a network. However, even the most rigidly devised organizational structure and process will not successfully contain all the inside and outside anxiety all of the time and, if it becomes overly pervasive and rigid, can even promote inside anxiety by foreclosing participation. Given the comforting aspects of institutionalized control and its accompanying rigidities, losses of accurate and timely reality testing, and creativity, intervention strategies must involve locating a level of institutionalization that still permits gathering good information about organizational performance as well as patient and payer expectations. Organization members must be constantly reminded that finding creative ways to adapt to changes in the rapidly evolving healthcare marketplace are essential to survival and that changing the rules and protocols may be necessary. These expectations may be modeled by appropriately challenging the way things have been traditionally done, which may challenge the current design of the organization and its work processes.

It must also be appreciated that structure and familiar process cannot be depended upon to accomplish everything. Dynamic leadership can often move things along after a reasonable level of consensus has developed over direction. As the case continues in the next section, the effects of forceful leadership can be observed.

Autocratic Group and Organizational Culture

The autocratic culture relieves member anxiety by promoting the belief among its members that a powerful, often charismatic, leader can control everything, including inside and outside anxiety. The leader, it is hoped, can save everyone from their problems and make them feel good. As a result, the leader ends up holding most of the power and can promote the correct behavior (as defined by the leader) that it is hoped will minimize everyone's anxiety, including that of the leader who fears being attacked as he or she fulfills his or her vision. Some members of the organization also fear attack by the leader because he or she often acts in ways that are at odds with their perspective. This tends to create alienated or disenfranchised employees who may try to strike back at anytime as individuals or as a group. At the same time, other members become the leader's favorites. Those who question the leader are scapegoated as troublemakers. Such interpersonal dynamics lead to divisiveness.

In addition, the charismatic leader may be found by organization members to be too human, a person who can exercise poor judgement, which is also distressing. Interpersonal rivalries spawned by access to the leader create conflict that disrupts work, which leads to the reemergence of inside anxiety. All of these outcomes lead to renewed inside anxiety.

The governing board or the majority of employees may eventually come to feel that replacing the leader is necessary; however, they also intuitively understand that this action is filled with the danger of being attacked by the leader and his or her followers. Feelings of guilt over challenging the leader may also be felt, further adding to the discomfort of making the change. It is at this juncture of increased anxiety and psychological defensiveness that a new leader may emerge to move the group to one of the other types.

The Case for Herd Behavior Many physicians prefer to have their medical groups led by a charismatic leader who is expected to take care of everything, thereby permitting them to focus their attention on the practice of medicine and, in academic health sciences centers, teaching and research.

Continuing with the case, once Dr. Fellow was ensconced as the leader responsible for developing the integration agreement, she quickly developed a kitchen cabinet of loyal followers who fed her information that supported her point of view. At the same time, outspoken critics of integration were targeted for discounting and scapegoating. They were gradually cut off from information and participation. Dr. Fellow also came to be known as a person who approved most requests related to the integration agreement if pressed. It was clear that she wanted to be liked and admired and that she would use the power of her role to grant requests to receive approval (the narcissistic response).

Gradually it became clear that, after consulting with her kitchen cabinet, Dr. Fellow was making all the major decisions regarding integration, which were then merely handed down to the members of GPC. Her one major concession was that she frequently met with Dr. Jones to keep him informed. The outcome of this process was that some group members became anxious about the direction of the changes Dr. Fellow was making (outside anxiety), but they felt helpless to make any changes (inside anxiety). No one was willing to oppose the now powerful Dr. Fellow and her in-group. As a result, GPC was torn apart by rivalry and dissention. Interpersonal and administrative wastelands developed where no one, including Dr. Fellow, was willing to venture. These outcomes eventually compromised the group's cohesion just when being able to act together was critically important. Many felt, including Dr. Jones, that at this key juncture performance was sufficiently threatened to merit another change in leadership. However, care had to be taken to not alienate Dr. Fellow and her faithful followers to avoid creating explosive and divisive group dynamics.

Case Analysis Powerful charismatic leaders can accomplish difficult tasks but often at a cost to long-term group cohesion, morale, and performance. In this case, making a change in leadership was going to be difficult. Dr. Jones had to take on a powerful leader who had built up a loyal following.

Intervention Strategy Autocratic leaders often end up making all of the decisions. This process makes them appear dedicated, overworked executives who assume personal responsibility for everything that happens. They are eventually willing if not forced (because of resistance to their direction) to micromanage just about every aspect of the organization and are willing to deal with anything brought to their attention. A by-product of their leadership style is the collection of a group of individuals (supporters) who are enamored of their power (narcissistic) and willing to support them no matter what (arrogant-vindictive).

Displacing an autocratic leader must, therefore, be regarded as no small risk. A common method is to elevate the person to a position with little formal power and authority and no access to resources. If accepted by the leader in question, this process of "kicking him or her upstairs" saves face, relieves him or her of the often punishing, self-imposed pressure he or she works under, while creating the space for a nondestructive organizational change.

A second strategy is to move the person to a similar role where his or her energies can be expended working on another problem area which, for the moment, needs strong leadership. A third strategy involves directly confronting the leader by asking the person to resign or face termination of his or her role. If the person involved has become highly dysfunctional and resistant to coaching and the authority of the CEO, this step may have to be taken (not unlike the celebrated confrontation between President Truman and General McArthur). This strategy is the most direct and efficient but also the most threatening, difficult, risky, and potentially painful one for a CEO to implement. This is the strategy that surfaces in the case as it continues in the next section.

A note should also be added about an ounce of prevention. Early intervention in the form of coaching by a member of the governing board, a consultant, or a former mentor can be successful in modifying a leader's tendency to assume the role of autocrat. These interventions do not work every time, but patience and persistence can be rewarded with change.

Intentional Group and Organizational Culture

Intentional group cultures, unlike the other three types of group cultures, are relatively free of inside and outside anxiety. Membership is not threatening, and there is little need for members to develop psychological, interpersonal, and social defenses against anxiety. The thoughts and feelings of individuals are respected. Conflicts are acknowledged and worked through. Consensus building works because it is accomplished in an open group dynamic where everyone feels his or her point of view is being heard. Working in the group is fun as well as challenging. Leadership of the group is often volunteered by members who have something to contribute, and their leadership efforts are accepted by others.

Intentional groups are threatened by the emergence of anxiety, which is now omnipresent in networks, hospitals, and medical groups dealing with a rapidly changing operating environment. Intentional groups may also be readily compromised by the emergence of leaders who strongly prefer one of the other three types of group or organizational cultures: homogenized, institutionalized, or autocratic. Their leadership emerges when sufficient anxiety develops. For example, a group member may vigorously point out that the cause of a problem is the lack of sufficient organization and that rules and regulations are being disregarded or should be developed. Another member may point out that the group needs a stronger, more visionary leader who can lead the group out of its current difficulties. There may also emerge a trend among some members to attack and disregard the contributions of other members. They may act without regard to direction offered by the group's leaders and those interested in continuing to work on the task. These tendencies are always present in groups and must be recognized and addressed (not suppressed) in order to maintain the intentional work group culture.

The Case for Ongoing Success Continuing with the case, Dr. Jones became exceedingly concerned that Dr. Fellow was going to prove to be a leader who was not ultimately able to build sufficient consensus, although it was clear she was in a position to ram the decision through. Dr. Jones decided to confront her over her inability to build consensus, and she recognized that the medical group was now seriously split. After discussing the situation, Dr. Fellow agreed that the best use of her talents was to return to her practice. She agreed to resign her role but not without protests from her group of supporters who made it clear that Dr. Jones was making a serious mistake and at a critical juncture. Dr. Jones subsequently announced he would assume personal responsibility for drawing the group together to work through an integration process. Despite having had to ask Dr. Fellow to step aside, Dr. Jones was highly admired and respected for his leadership and management abilities. He immediately set about developing a new leadership group that included many of Dr. Fellow's key people. He also hired a consultant to facilitate the group's work toward building consensus. There gradually evolved under his leadership a collaborative camaraderie that eventually produced a successful merger with MHCS.

Case Analysis Making any group as successful as possible requires gaining the creativity and productivity of all its members. Intentional group dynamics tap this potential the best of any of the groups. Individual autonomy is respected which reduces anxiety for those who are concerned about their independence. Appropriate levels of rules, regulations, and policies are present and enforced, which reduces anxiety for those who like a lot of structure. However, rigidity is avoided by constantly questioning their applicability to accomplishing work. The intentional group and organizational culture also provide opportunities for others to lead and explore their leadership capabilities. At the same time, there always exists the tendency for the group or organizational culture to gravitate to one of the other three types of culture.

Intervening in Group and Organizational Culture

Informed interventions must begin with an understanding of the current culture. The above four types of group cultures are readily spotted as are tendencies to develop a second group culture in response to problems of the dominant culture of the moment. Once an understanding is developed, an effort may be made to move the group toward greater intentionality by making the current situation unacceptable and, therefore, stressful and by avoiding fight/flight tendencies to bolt to another dysfunctional group culture. A healthcare or physician executive responsible for coaching the change must be sensitive to the seductiveness of the three dysfunctional group cultures and to the constant pressure exerted by some members to lead the group in their direction. A constant press of explanation, expectations, and rewards for change are most effective in leading organizational change. Ordering change, restructuring, hiring new managers, replacing employees, and reducing the workforce, while affecting the culture and perhaps destroying it, often only encourage the strong reemergence of psychologically defensive thoughts, feelings, and actions and the development of defensive group cultures.

Movement in the direction of intentionality can, as discussed in Chapter 9, also be facilitated by education about group process and by using staff trained in group process consultation. Difficult transitions can also be facilitated by consultants experienced in facilitating change.

In sum, intervening in group culture requires insight into organizational and group dynamics and the knowledge and skills to facilitate intentional work. Every aspect of an intervention includes many contingencies, some that may be foreseen and some that may not be. An executive who must lead change toward intentional work must be persistent and patient. He or she must also be prepared to create stress that results in anxiety and that in turn motivates a change in group culture. At the same time, group members must receive sincere caretaking attention and respect, and they must learn they are trusted. These actions on the part of a healthcare or physician executive model behavior, thoughts, and feelings that direct attention toward the intentional group culture where everyone is respected and trusted and where empowerment exists and the generation of new ideas and the taking of risks is rewarded rather than punished. Executives may also be aided in their work by psychologically informed group and organizational process consultants who are experienced in facilitating cultural change.

Conclusion

There is much to understand about group and organizational dynamics, which are often driven by their members' wish to avoid anxiety. The four groups discussed illustrate that group dynamics are always present. Understanding group dynamics does not mean that the leader, a group member, or someone outside of the group can easily change group dynamics. Each of the three types of psychologically defensive, potentially dysfunctional groups offers its members relief from anxiety; and so long as it fulfills this purpose, changing the group dynamic is difficult. However, when anxiety reemerges, as a result of overwhelming internal or external pressure, it is likely the culture will change. The group will renew its efforts to make the current group type work better, or it will change to one of the other types of groups. Appreciating this enables those responsible for organizational and subgroup performance to be prepared to facilitate or direct changes to the group's dynamics.

Endnote

1. This chapter is informed by the work of Edgar H. Schein, *Organizational Culture and Leadership* (San Francisco: Jossey-Basy, 1985); Michael A. Diamond and Seth Allcorn, "The Psychodynamics of Regression in Work Groups," *Human Relations,* 40 (August 1987): 8, 525–543; Seth Allcorn, "Understanding Groups at Work," *Personnel,* 66 (August 1981): 8, 28–36; and the notion of organizational identity developed by Michael Diamond, *The Unconscious Life of Organizations: Interpreting Organizational Identity* (Westport CT: Quorum, 1993).

CHAPTER 6

DEFENSIVE HOSPITAL AND MEDICAL GROUP CULTURES

Working together effectively in groups has always been important and has become even more important as hospitals have implemented management techniques such as TQM, downsizing, and reengineering and as medical groups have become larger and more complex. The rapidly changing and stressful nature of the healthcare marketplace places hospitals and medical groups, and by extension the groups that operate them, under ever-increasing pressure, which produces many anxieties and accompanying psychologically defensive group cultures. Anxieties are also increased by the need to plan and implement change within hospitals and medical groups.

Chapter 5 introduced the three psychologically defensive group and organization cultures and the intentional nondefensive culture. A mix of hospital and medical group case examples were provided. This chapter provides additional examples of psychologically defensive group processes by focusing on the two fundamental, constituent parts of networks: hospitals and medical groups. Each of the four types of group and organizational cultures is explained, and case examples are provided for first hospitals and then medical groups. Intervention strategies are suggested for each case example.

Working Together in Groups in Hospitals

Group process and culture help to defend members against anxiety and provide answers to questions of what the group is;

145

how it works; and how members are to think, feel, and act. The following discussion uses the homogenized, institutionalized, and autocratic group and organizational cultures to explore work life in hospitals.[1]

Homogenized Hospital Group and Organizational Culture

This group or organizational culture is not common in hospitals that have relatively clear organizational structures; however, when desires for autonomy and independence emerge, this group culture arises even in the most tightly organized and controlled of hospitals. Homogenized group process discourages leadership because there is no followership. Members of homogenized groups experience their lack of connectedness and relatedness to each other as threatening, especially when significant organizational stress develops. When the going gets tough, the lack of connectedness and followership plunges the group into difficulty with coordinating work on its tasks. Group experience becomes threatening, and safety is sought. Leading seems dangerous, as does following. Individual flight from these conditions and accompanying anxiety is natural. Under these circumstances, withdrawing physically and psychologically becomes one of the safest things to do. Employees may also seek support and safety from others. And, as noted in Chapter 5, if the group's members feel sufficiently threatened, a switch may occur to one of the other types of groups.

A homogenized group arose in a hospital when a committee was created and charged with resolving a number of problems involving missing and late medical record documentation and medical record completion after discharge. Laboratory tests were often missing or misfiled as were occasional reports from radiology, physical therapy, and other ancillary services. Physicians often did not complete records at the time of discharge, and many were reluctant to come to the medical records department to clear up deficiencies. The committee included staff from many areas in the hospital as well as several physicians. Committee members eventually identified dozens of major problems that had to be resolved in order for the committee to fulfill its mission. It is noteworthy that some of the problems had been around for years and that other committees had worked on them without success. The committee's progress gradually slowed to a near stop within a few months because its members resisted returning to their respective departments to solve the problems that were creating the missing medical record documentation. The physician committee members were equally resistant to confronting their colleagues over their behavior. Gradually, committee members became critical of each other and stopped listening to each other during committee meetings. Attendance fell off, and it became clear that the committee would accomplish little else, although it continued meeting occasionally to review its lack of progress.

Intervention Strategy Committees that work on sweeping problems, some of which have been around for many years and are known to require investments in new technology or a major change in management style or attitude on the part of a few key individuals, need to have a senior level executive as a chair or at the minimum as a member to insure that members feel empowered to take on the tough problems. Subcommittees or total quality management committees might also be formed around some of the discovered problems. The committee should also be encouraged to designate strategies for resolution, including a time line for resolution, and to provide adequate resources to do its work.

Institutionalized Hospital Group and Organizational Culture

This is a much more common group culture in hospitals. This culture defends its members from anxiety by providing rules, regulations, and formal roles that control many of the employees' interactions. These rules are often codified in the hospital policies and procedures manual. Everyone is supposed to know what to think, feel, and do, and what others are to think, feel, and do, and they must know the procedures by which work is to be accomplished. The process often includes focusing decision making at the top. This group culture accomplishes work but at the cost of creativity, flexibility, and the opportunity to learn from experience.

It is noteworthy that hospitals have historically had difficulty adjusting to the rapidly changing healthcare delivery marketplace, which may well be a symptom of excessive institutionalization. Resistance to change energizes self-interest, organizational politics, self-protection, special interest groups, and power plays that disrupt planned changes. Caregivers also abhor the accompanying rigidities, restrictions, and paperwork, which do not always yield the expected outcomes. These eventualities, when combined with a lack of flexibility and poor organizational learning, end up threatening the long-term viability of hospitals. If the perceived threat to a department or hospital is great enough, it can result in a migration to another type of group culture.

An example of an institutionalized process is budgeting. Hospital budgeting processes often include many rules about performing the work as well as many top-down requests and expectations. Budgeting can become an exceptionally time-consuming and onerous task that is resisted by those who do not understand all of the complexity or see how it relates to the hospital's caregiving mission. Budgeting is also often accompanied by variance reporting (sometimes monthly) as well as many ad hoc questions and requests for additional research, including detailed review and evaluation of major purchases. Work on the budget can seem like the only thing that matters even though it is a numerical abstraction of what is actually occurring in the hospital.

Intervention Strategy Institutionalized processes that contain a lot of rules and that are often controlled from the top have their place in hospitals; however, when the rules and control take on a significance greater than their true value, employees become alienated and morale and work suffer. Executives and employ- ees must feel comfortable in speaking out when the balance between rules and controls, and work seems to have shifted toward the former. This is not, however, always the case be- cause changing the rules, controls, and processes often appear to be the sacred privilege of an elite few and, therefore, potentially too threatening to challenge. The CEO and senior-level execu- tives should be encouraged to meet one-on-one with managers throughout the hospital to learn their thoughts and feelings about how the hospital is being run. Focus groups may also be valu- able as well as a visit from a consultant trained to gather quali- tative information from employees and managers for feedback to top management. Work and processes that become rigidly institutionalized and, therefore, cannot be questioned must be questioned; otherwise, the hospital assumes the additional risk of not being adaptive.

Autocratic Hospital Group and Organizational Culture

The autocratic group culture is also common in hospitals. It is not uncommon to find a CEO who makes, or at the minimum endorses, all major decisions and sometimes even minor ones. Other hospital executives and managers are also expected to exercise high levels of control over subordinates and their work. These executives and managers are expected to take charge, which rules out employees assuming personal responsibility for the hospital's success. These executives can end up dominating subordinates with the tacit collusion of many of those being led. As a result, a few executives and physicians end up holding most of the power. In- and out-groups develop, and those who question what is going on are scapegoated as troublemakers. These interpersonal dynamics lead to divisiveness and rivalry and competition for access to the CEO, which disrupts work and leads to frequent outbreaks of anxiety arising from the rumor of the day. The CEO can also become disconnected from the nature of the hospital's operations, which can eventually lead to a change to another group culture.

Autocratic group culture can arise when the CEO suddenly decides to engage in downsizing and reengineering in response to a fall in the hospital's census. Although virtually all senior-level executives, department heads, and employees understand that the hospital must adjust to the reduced census, they are not consulted regarding this momentous decision. The CEO decides to hire a major consulting company noted for downsizing and reengineering hospitals. Most executives do not agree with this approach; however, the CEO insists. The CEO makes all of the decisions regarding which firm to hire and the scope of their work and also takes the position that he must approve all open positions in order to achieve some immediate downsizing through attrition. Senior level executives and department heads begin to feel cut off from participating and ineffective. After the consulting engagement begins, the CEO gradually withdraws from participating in meetings, preferring to rely on the advice of the consulting company, which includes providing employees a slick program of communication about the "rightsizing," which further closes off the opportunity for free and open discussion of events.

Intervention Strategy Autocratic unilateral actions on the part of CEOs and other powerful executives are fairly common in hospitals. Participative or more collaborative management styles should be considered by those in charge and if necessary encouraged by the governing board if the CEO is highly autocratic. Constant reliance on autocratic and paternalistic or maternalistic methods promotes uncertainty and dependence as well as discounting what everyone else in the hospital has to contribute. Training programs that focus on team building and collaboration as well as the use of consultants trained in interpersonal, group, and organizational dynamics will also be beneficial. Total quality management principles are yet another avenue of pursuit consistent with promoting open participation and reflective work processes and collaborative leadership styles. Discussion of the culture of groups within hospitals and of the hospital as a whole leads to similar discussion concerning medical groups.

Working Together in Groups in Medical Group Practice

Understanding group process is especially helpful to better understanding how medical groups operate. The three types of common, but in part dysfunctional, group types introduced in Chapter 5 contribute to understanding medical group organizational dynamics.

Homogenized Medical Group and Organizational Culture

This group culture is especially likely to be found in medical groups where the principals of the medical group—the physicians—are often keenly interested in maintaining personal autonomy and independence. The result is that management of their groups can be difficult. Examples of problems in medical group governance are common. A colleague once reported that, while he was being interviewed as a candidate to manage a medical group, he inquired about the group's decision-making process. He was told the group had over 50 physicians, and often had to agree or no decision could be made. This story epitomizes the nature of a homogenized group culture. Everyone has to be treated the same, even if at times the group's success is compromised in the process. These same dynamics can occur in virtually any subgroup or committee of a larger group where everyone appears to hold veto power. Compromised decision making and lack of change can, however, eventually lead to the group feeling threatened as competitors succeed in invading the group's catchment area and managed care contracting fails at key points.

Intervention Strategy The tendency of physicians to see each other as equals and colleagues, and their often negative experience of administrators who often resort to uses of power and authority that result in resistance to their leadership are major influences that consistently produce homogenized group and subgroup cultures. Countervailing these often omnipresent tendencies can become one of the primary tasks of leading the group and its members as well as managing the group's activities. Recognizing that these tendencies exist; appreciating their origins, which are in part associated with the selection of a profession that has autonomy; understanding how physicians are socialized to know themselves and their work; and, most importantly, accepting and respecting these tendencies are the first steps in being able to successfully lead and manage in the pervasive presence of the homogenization that these tendencies create. If hospital or physician executives see these tendencies as merely bad and off-task, unresolvable conflict is likely to result, as the physicians will not abandon their value systems and views about executives and administrators.

Knowing and accepting these tendencies in physicians promotes the ability to work together even though the tendencies make time-consuming consensus building necessary. A number of more traditional management actions can also minimize the adverse effects of these tendencies. The nature of leadership and management roles must be described, explained, and as nearly as possible, agreed to among all members. Physician and medical group executives must also make every effort to work openly and maintain good communications with all members of the group. Considerable ambiguity must be tolerated as well as the delays that inevitably develop as an effort is made to build a consensus around major decisions. Consensus as used here implies everyone's point of view is heard but not necessarily agreed to. Patience is also a virtue, because even after maximum communication, education, and participation, implementation of an agreed-to-plan may be challenged by some physicians and not understood by others.

Institutionalized Medical Group and Organizational Culture

This culture is less common in medical groups with members who are resistant to rules and paperwork, if not adamantly opposed to them. At the same time, physicians expect the group to operate effortlessly at low cost and to meet all of their needs as well as those of their patients. This, of course, is often only accomplished with some institutionalization of work processes and routine decision making, which inevitably contains expectations that the physicians will comply with some rules and regulations and, for example, complete their medical records and other forms as requested. Those responsible for maintaining the daily operations of medical groups must be sensitive to striking a balance between what is perceived to be a bureaucratic process and the need to get legitimate work done. It is often easy to find some medical group members who hold as one of their higher achievements finding ways to circumvent operating rules. At other times, some physicians may be infuriated about the rules, loudly complain, and threaten to leave the group.

Examples abound. Some physicians consistently do not complete their medical records. Others periodically give staff erroneous instructions or cut special deals that violate procedures and occasionally the law. An example of this type of disdain and disregard for necessary procedure occurred when Dr. Jeckle hired his sister's daughter as his secretary. Barbara was told to report to work on a Monday, and Dr. Jeckle provided her with the desk of a recently departed secretary who, the leadership of the medical group had decided, was not going to be replaced, at least in the near future. Barbara worked diligently at her first full-time job for six weeks before she finally phoned the personnel administrator to inquire about when she would receive her first pay check. Her presence in the medical group of course, was news to the administrator who had not been informed. Barbara was placed on the payroll and the situation reviewed at length by the senior management of the medical group. The group did not have the resources to continue paying her, and the medical group's policy on nepotism had also been violated. It was also clear that Dr. Jeckle's blatant disregard for the medical group's policies and rules had infuriated a number of other employees.

Toward the end of the period of review, Dr. Jeckle began to make increasing demands on Barbara to perform work not related to her job, such as purchasing gifts for his family members and dropping his car off for repairs. When she declined to take his dog to the vet, he blew up and fired her on the spot without consulting the personnel administrator. She almost immediately obtained an attorney (her father was one), and an out-of-court settlement was eventually reached.

Intervention Strategy The tendency of physicians and, with their encouragement, some staff to resist conforming to needed and often agreed-to polices and procedures and rules and regulations is present in most medical groups. The aggravation experienced often leads to outspoken objection to, denigration of, disregard for, circumvention of, and even personal attacks upon those trying to do their job by either following the policies and procedures or trying to enforce them. Once again, it is important to appreciate that some physicians and staff are adamantly opposed to being controlled, monitored, and regulated and find these inevitabilities coercive and unacceptable. Patience and persistence are, therefore, demanded as well as tolerance of nonconformity even after the best efforts to enlist the offender's goodwill and cooperation.

Explaining why the institutionalized processes exist can sometimes helps. For example, in the above case, Dr. Jeckle learned very quickly about proper hiring procedure if people were going to get paid and proper termination procedure if lawsuits were to be avoided. This latter point was further driven home by deducting the amount of the settlement from his income. However, despite the best efforts to communicate and educate, physicians often either avoid trying to understand or simply do not have a frame of reference to understand and appreciate why the policies and procedures are necessary. Orientations and hands-on demonstrations of how they work can help. Participation in groups and committees responsible for developing and revising policies and procedures can also be illuminating and can elicit their cooperation. However, in the end, disciplinary measures must also be considered, including threatened losses of income through linkages of earnings to compliance, fines, and even termination.

Autocratic Medical Group and Organizational Culture

The autocratic group culture is not uncommon to medical groups despite the tendency of their members to avoid being directly controlled or subordinated. Many physicians prefer to be left alone to practice medicine. They accept that they have to play by institutional rules most of the time and that someone must lead and manage the group so long as whatever is done does not adversely affect their practice, working relationships, or income. Given this attitude, many physicians are more than happy to wash their hands of any participation in management of their group.

This tendency became abundantly clear during a meeting of the heads of the many subspecialties of an academic department in a school of medicine. The department chairman at the time had mismanaged the department's resources by promising everyone who asked for a resource that resource (narcissistic style). The department was overextended and beginning to run a deficit. During a meeting, the chairman, to his credit, admitted to the problems. The heads of the subspecialties were then asked to indicate their preference along a continuum for the type of leadership style they preferred. A line was drawn on a board anchored at one end by the notion that the chairman would make most of the decision and at the other end by a participative approach that would involve them in decision making. Despite the major problems the department was experiencing due to the many unilateral and unsound decisions the chairman had made, nine out of ten of those present selected the autocratic end of the leadership spectrum. They just simply had enough to do and did not want to become involved in participating more actively in how the department was run. As a result, the chairman felt fully empowered to continue his methods, and the department's decline continued.

Intervention Strategy An autocratic group culture can readily emerge and, once established, is difficult to change. Those in power like it; those opposed have left or given up; and so long as those in charge do not create too many problems, the rest who just want to be left alone do not care. The result is that no top-down intervention will occur. Change will usually occur only if a sufficient number of medical group members are willing to openly act. This may occur if senior-level positions are voted on or if medical group members make it clear that change is expected and that the current physician executive(s) must step down. This is most likely to occur when most members of the medical group understand it is in serious trouble and that a change in leadership is necessary. Short of change, there are some things members can do if the autocratic culture becomes too dominant. Members can ask to participate in committees to consider major decisions rather than have those in power make them with a minimum of consultation with medical group members and employees. Instances of special favoritism and marginal decisions may be confronted in person, in writing, or possibly in meetings. Challenging those in authority, however, is a risky venture in that the challengers are likely to labeled dissenters and not team players. Change below the level of the CEO, however, can occur through his or her intervention. A subgroup or committee that develops an autocratic group culture that becomes dysfunctional can be changed by reorganizing the subgroup or committee, changing or reassigning its leaders to others tasks, or possibly even eliminating the committee.

Conclusion

This chapter explained and elaborated on the importance of understanding the psychologically defensive aspects of group and organizational cultures of the hospitals and medical groups that must be successfully combined to create comprehensive, full-service, healthcare delivery networks. The examples, problems, and intervention strategies point the way toward dealing with psychologically defensive group and organizational processes. Chapters 7 and 8 will focus on the significance of psychologically defensive individual and group dynamics because they form the underlying bases for the development of group and organizational philosophies which direct thinking, feeling and action, and the development of organizational culture.

Endnote

1. This chapter is informed by the work of Edgar H. Stein, *Organizational Culture and Leadership* (San Francisco: Jossey-Bass, 1985); Michael A. Diamond and Seth Allcorn, "The Psychodynamics of Regression in Work Groups," *Human Relations,* 40 (August 1987): 525–543; and Seth Allcorn, "Understanding Groups at Work," *Personnel,* 66 (August, 1989): 28–36.

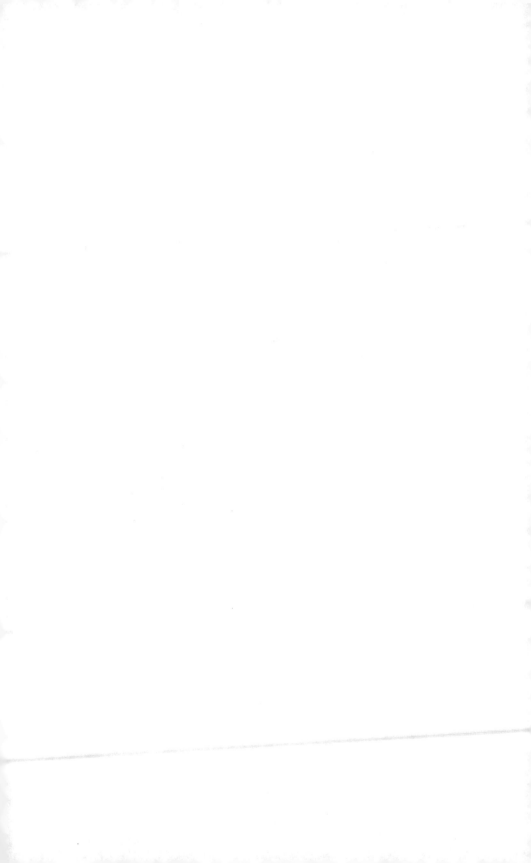

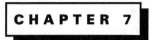

CHAPTER 7

THE FOUNDATION
OF NETWORK CULTURE

This chapter further explores the importance of interpersonal, group, and organizational dynamics by taking an in-depth look at the philosophical side of networks, hospitals, and medical groups. The development of a large, fully integrated, regional healthcare delivery network must be accompanied by the creation of an overarching culture containing basic assumptions about life, others, and work (workplace philosophies). Network executives are responsible for allaying anxieties and for creating an overall direction for the development of workplace philosophies, and by extension, their organization's culture.

We are, however, reminded by the preceding chapters of this book that many aspects of organizational life are not readily subjected to management and are often not even readily known to exist by the members of an organization. These considerations return us to the psychological, interpersonal, and group nature of organizational life where many aspects of the organization are shared among its members as subconscious content. This content is the basis for many of the philosophies that become part of the building blocks of organizational culture.

In this book, the linkage of unconscious processes such as psychological defenses; the development of out-of-awareness but shared basic assumptions about the nature of life, others, organizations, and work; and their translation into workplace philosophies that are not always stated but nonetheless influential, brings with it a note of caution. It must be appreciated that under stressful conditions, psychological defenses tend to distort perception of

159

what is, how people are, and how work is accomplished. Psychological defenses such as rationalization and denial can change reality into something more acceptable or entirely block it out. Other types of psychological defenses deaden experience or lead to seeing people and actions as black and white, all good or all bad. These outcomes often occur when stress and anxiety increase, just when clear thinking and accurate reality testing are critical to success.

The result is that the basic assumptions themselves become warped and disconnected from reality. This creates the basis for a group and organizational culture that contains social pathology, which in turn promotes more anxiety and psychological defensiveness, which usually reinforces the preexisting psychological defenses, and by extension, the underlying philosophies of the group and organizational culture. This must be kept in mind when management and consultants offer the often well-deserved observation that there is something fundamentally wrong that makes a hospital, medical group, or other organization dysfunctional. It is equally important to appreciate that it is from the unconsciously held and often aggressively defended psychological defenses and assumptions that much of the resistance to change arises.

In sum, changing management and leadership styles and group and organizational dynamics must not be taken as a mere exercise in management prerogative. Those who are able to successfully manage cultural change and transformation are those who will be able to comprehend many of the psychologically defensive elements of existing group and organizational dynamics before working to create change.

This chapter recasts and expands the discussion of the unconscious side of organizational life and accompanying basic assumptions that contribute to the development of workplace philosophies and culture discussed in Chapters 5 and 6 to a discussion of the philosophical nature of organizational life. This side of organizational life is not often given much thought although it contains the substance of what makes organizations tick and what allays anxiety about work life.[1] In this regard, the philosophical nature of organizations is another way to understand the effects of workplace anxieties and accompanying psychological defenses. Workplace philosophies are, in part, a product of these unconscious dynamics. This chapter continues by discussing some of the important attributes leaders must have to be successful in leading organizational and cultural change.

The Underlying Philosophical Assumptions of Organizational Culture

Management is much more than the science of finding the most cost-effective way to produce a service. Everyone who works holds unacknowledged assumptions about nature, people, work, reality, and relationships. These assumptions, in many hard-to-detect ways, are also constantly influenced by executives. Understanding them informs healthcare and physician executives at a fundamental level that permits them to see work life and its many emotional and hard-to-identify properties clearly enough to endeavor to change them. Changing culture, therefore, begins with understanding these attributes of the current culture, mapping out the desired cultural elements and then developing interventions that facilitate transition to the philosophical underpinnings of the new culture. It does not begin with announcing that a change in organizational culture is desirable and will now be implemented. This naive view of organizational culture and cultural change, however, occurs all too often and always with predictable results: no change.

Changing culture takes insight, care, and many years of patient work. Total quality management (TQM) is a good example of one aspect of organizational culture that is embraced by many hospitals. Its proponents speak of its implementation taking years even when it receives the constant support of senior management. TQM is also an example of a type of cultural change that implies a transformation in how organization members understand the world, organization, processes, themselves, others, and work.

The Nature of the World of the Network

Understanding the world around us translates into knowing who we are. We must also be able to differentiate the various organizations that compose the network and be able to tell the network from other networks and providers. Understanding the nature of a network's many organizational parts and how they fit together to create a whole is important for employees and executives in order for them to adjust their thoughts, feelings, and actions to better fit what the network is and is doing. For example, the acquisition of a major new primary care physician group that is not immediately communicated to the rest of the networked organizations and employees can lead to confusion, unintentional undermining, and even anger about not being informed on a more timely and perhaps complete basis.

Understanding where the network ends and the rest of the world begins is equally important. Executives and employees must understand the geographic boundaries of the network, what organizations it relates to, and who its competitors are in order to be effective contributors to its well-being.

The creation of a sense of wholeness is not easily accomplished in healthcare delivery networks. Employee awareness and loyalty rest with their hospital, medical group, or related service organization. Merely legal combining of these organizations creates little awareness of a greater whole. This lack of common awareness can ultimately compromise the success of the network by frustrating its ability to function as a whole and provide seamless healthcare delivery. Every effort must be made to clarify to employees what the network is and its overall mission. Executives should be hired or committees established to insure the meaningful development of a common sense of the network and its culture.

A second aspect of the nature of networks is the beliefs and assumptions held by executives and employees about the nature of the network. These beliefs and assumptions can be highly informed and realistic, or they can suffer from some degree of personal and group psychological disorganization. Basic beliefs about a network can become disorienting and nonadaptive when its leaders hold unrealistic beliefs about themselves, others, the network, and the world. Network employees end up living and working in a setting that increases their anxieties rather than allaying them. Increased anxiety provokes the use of reality-distorting psychological defenses rather than discouraging them. The basic assumptions that network executives hold about the nature of the network are, therefore, critically important and should be open to self-reflection and examination by others. If an executive feels that the world is filled with threat, he or she will feel that threat exists everywhere and his or her often unfounded fears will govern decision making and work.

Human Nature

Beliefs about our nature and the nature of others are often unwittingly based on what we have learned from life experience. A healthcare or physician executive who believes that people are lazy, untrustworthy, inconsiderate, unthinking, and unpredictable will also feel they have to be constantly watched and motivated to work. These beliefs may also be held for certain types of people or groups of people and for specific aspects of an organization.

An opposite set of beliefs is that people are inherently "good," trustworthy, thoughtful, and hard working, and that organizations are socially conscious and contribute to making the world a better place. It is likely that all of these beliefs are held. Which ones emerge depends on recent experience, current state of mind, and the situation. Once again, the assumptions we hold about the nature of ourselves, others, and organizations come full circle to the unconscious influence of our thoughts and feelings.

Healthcare and physician executives leading the development of and managing large integrated healthcare delivery networks must constantly examine their assumptions about human nature in order to remain grounded in reality. A particularly important aspect of remaining reflective deals with the assumptions made about the nature of the organizations being incorporated into the integration effort. Many disruptive and potentially destructive and unfounded assumptions may be held, such as viewing a newly integrated hospital as deficient and needing to be whipped into shape. This may result in immediately and prematurely moving to downsize and reorganize it. Care must be taken to learn about the hospital, its culture, its employees, its services, and what makes it tick before making major changes. This process of getting to know a networked organization can prevent false assumptions about its nature that either encourage changing it because it is thought to be bad in some way or emulate it because it is thought to be good.

The Nature of Work

We all hold beliefs about the nature of our actions relative to others and the world. We might see ourselves and our organization as powerful and instrumental, or we might see ourselves and our organization as helpless, dependent, and ineffective, unable to take action, or only able to react to change. Depending upon which beliefs are held, the leaders and members of a networked organization may feel that their work is important or they may feel that they are ineffective and that their labors accomplish little. Healthcare and physician-executives may also feel helpless and look to collecting more and more information in the hope that it will make the decision for them. Or perhaps they do nothing, hoping that if they wait to see what will happen, the problem will go away.

Influences such as these dominate healthcare delivery organizations where these conservative and risk-aversive assumptions about work and personal effectiveness exist along a continuum from feeling valued and influential to frustrated and helpless. How the leaders of networks feel about themselves and their organization is the critical variable in how caregivers and other employees come to understand themselves, each other, their work, and the network.

Healthcare and physician executives responsible for developing an integrated network of providers must also take the time to learn about the beliefs of the executives of the organizations that become integrated. All healthcare organization executives differ in their beliefs, which may make them more or less receptive to integration and change. They may steadfastly see themselves as visionary and autonomous and, therefore, unwilling to accept subordination. Their beliefs may also make them overly eager to become integrated in the hope of being saved. Network executives must be sensitive to these beliefs about work and personal effectiveness in order to make their network's integrated parts achieve optimal performance.

The Nature of the Network's Reality

Understanding the facts can be difficult. Often, the facts used to make network, hospital, and medical group decisions are not necessarily based on hard evidence or the input of stakeholders who will be affected by the decision. Typically, leaders of large organizations base many decisions on subjective processes, experiences, and layers of filtered analyses and reports that can conceal hidden agendas. Decision making can be dominated by the personal biases of a few powerful people at the top. These considerations raise concerns about the nature of organizational knowledge and rationality. Healthcare and physician executives must be careful about what they think is true. Subjective reality must not take over even if it conveniently supports one's views or appears to readily solve a problem.

Reality is hard to know in a large, complex, fully-integrated healthcare delivery network. The network will inevitably include many layers through which information must be passed as well as a broad spectrum of horizontal communications and relationships that can ultimately make its nature and what is going on

165

virtually unknowable. Network executives must be exceptionally careful about developing an alternate view of reality that is out of touch with the true complexity of their organization and what is happening to it and within it. It becomes incredibly easy to make misguided decisions based on incomplete, inaccurate, and unrepresentative information when the pressure of having to constantly change is factored in. It should be noted that total quality management principles encourage the development of objective data for decision making.

The Nature of Human Relations in Networks

Network employees may hold many different assumptions about what constitutes a suitable interpersonal relationship. Workplace relationships raise the issues of autonomy and control. Relating to powerful superiors can be threatening and infantalizing if their behavior is autocratic, paternalistic, manipulative, and controlling. Relationships can also be liberating where meaningful delegation, empowerment, participation, trust, and respect exist. How relationships are imposed from above and reacted to from below are often dominated by unconscious processes that can lead to unproductive working relationships. Healthcare and physician executives must be sensitive to how their actions affect others.

Network executives must be exceptionally sensitive to those who operate the many different organizations that compose the network as well as the network's many different functions. Considerable effort will be required to avoid being seen as autocratic. The network may only survive and prosper as a result of vigorous leadership efforts to build consensus.

The nature of the world, human nature, work, reality, and working together contain the basic organizational cultural assumptions that are hard to detect, question, and change. Their management, however, is a critical aspect of achieving excellence. Executives responsible for developing large integrated networks of providers will have to frequently deal with the need to lead the work of organizational cultural change.

Leading Organizational Cultural Change

Network, hospital, and medical group cultures are, for the most part, so omnipresent and in many ways unobserved that they are seldom understood to be present or to have a major influence on how organization members experience their workplace. The culture is essentially taken for granted. However, its unseen nature does not detract from its ability to minimize the experience of anxiety for organization members by making work life more predictable, less complex, and less threatening.

Organizational culture weaves history and myths, processes, ideas, and philosophies together to make things predictable and help members feel they belong while preventing their feeling they are being controlled by the organization. Organizational culture provides a meaning that is shared by organization members that, if disturbed, creates anxiety that spawns resistance to change. In the final analysis, organizational culture is the well-worn path for thinking and feeling about work that is often unacknowledged but includes basic assumptions about ourselves, others, and the work world.

Based on this understanding of organizational culture, changing it is predictably threatening. Interventions create anxiety as the old ways of thinking and feeling are openly challenged and new and unfamiliar ways are put forward to replace them. Network, hospital, and medical group members are asked to exchange what is familiar and safe for something new and different. And they have to at least temporarily work harder to create the change.

Network, hospital, and medical group employees quickly come to understand that they have to (1) learn something new, (2) work through a period of transition from the old ways to the new ways, (3) work out and perfect the new ways, (4) cope with their fear that they cannot learn the new ways, and (5) cope with their shame about how it was they let their old systems fail. They must do more work for an extended period of time. They must also work through their anxieties, fears, shame, and anger, and they must work through planning and implementing the change while keeping the network, hospital, and medical group running. That this is a lot to ask of anyone must be appreciated by healthcare and physician executives leading cultural change.

Network, hospital, and medical group leaders can help their employees work through their feelings and work harder to make the needed changes. This helping requires them to have a clear direction for the change, communicate it to organization members, and then point the way toward making the change. They must be prepared to be standfast in the storm of problems and difficulties that inevitably accompany change. They must hold high expectations, but they must also be prepared to bandage the knees of employees who fall along the way. If healthcare and physician executives sincerely care; point to the way through uncertainty; coach, coax, and prod a little along the way; and reward and celebrate successes while minimizing the finding of fault, they will hold the people of the organization together. This type of environment helps contain the fears and anxieties and absorb or deflect the anger of organization members while providing a caring and nurturing environment where making change is safe.

These are indeed weighty responsibilities for healthcare and physician executives to assume. Assuming them is facilitated by the following leadership attributes that support cultural change.

Objectivity

Healthcare and physician executives who lead cultural change must be objective and intentional even though the network, hospital, and medical group becomes awash in a sea of conflicting feelings and distorted thinking. Care must be taken to collect accurate and representative information as well as interpret and use it to manage change. Maintaining objectivity is aided by keen insights into the dynamics of the group culture of the network, hospital, and medical group; the nature of change; and the powerful effects they have upon how leaders experience themselves, the organization, and its members. Healthcare and physician executives must be able to sort out the important from the unimportant, and they must be able to prioritize problem solving with a certainty that reassures others. However, they should not feel they must make all the decisions. The preferred method is to include all levels of management in setting direction, establishing priorities, and designing change to establish a sense of empowerment through ownership of the change process.

Challenging Culture

Healthcare and physician executives must be willing to challenge, break down, and unfreeze (but not necessarily refreeze) the current culture, which will be experienced by its members as disorienting and anxiety producing. This is often a solitary task to which many of those in the organizational roles may eventually be recruited. The need for change must be communicated without alienating network, hospital, and medical group members who may consciously or unconsciously collude to block and reject the change. Healthcare and physician executives must also be willing to put the interests of the network, hospital, and medical group before personal needs to be accepted and admired. This altruistic act is an essential aspect of leading a shift in organizational culture. However, by making the sacrifice, feelings of compassion are encouraged in others while they are making what may feel to them like a long, and difficult journey that will tax their courage.

Inner Strength

Healthcare and physician executives must possess enough inner strength to withstand the many stresses and anxieties that will develop as organization members become fearful, angry, confused, uncertain, and resistant. They must have a realistic and strong sense of self-esteem that minimizes their anxiety and enables them to resist becoming personally disorganized and doubtful when major problems are encountered. Leaders of cultural change must accept that they will become the targets of anger and aggression. They must also be prepared to persist with their effort while remaining caring and understanding. They must above all else avoid the temptation to attack those who are resistant, which will only reassure them that they have been right and righteous for resisting. A constant show of support and confidence by governing board members and CEOs is a prerequisite for successful cultural change.

Inspiration

Healthcare and physician executives must be able to lead organization members to a new set of basic assumptions that are artfully developed and inspirationally presented. They must also model the new assumptions by paying attention to those aspects of organizational life that the change emphasizes. They are carefully watched, and the appearance of double standards and inconsistencies can be depended upon to detract from cultural change.

Participation

Healthcare and physician executives must allow for meaningful participation, including delegating and empowering subordinates to create change. They must be a good listeners and willing to work alongside those experiencing the change. Everyone must be enlisted in the change effort by the leaders.

Dealing with the Symbolic

Healthcare and physician executives must be effective at dealing with the symbolic. They must be able to understand the meaning of the old basic assumptions and how they are symbolized in order to be effective at removing them and replacing them with a new set of assumptions and symbols. Terminating a much loved and respected elderly physician for not meeting new standards of productivity can be a serious mistake in managing the symbolic nature of a newly integrated medical group, just as imposing a new physician executive on the group might be. Symbols are important and must be discovered and respected. They can be removed, changed, and substituted but only with care.

Conclusion

This chapter has built upon all of the previous chapters to explain the critically important aspects of often unacknowledged philosophical elements of networks, hospitals, and medical groups. They are very real and provide comforting direction and meaning, which minimizes anxiety and psychologically defensive responses to organizational life. It is these familiar, directing, and comforting aspects of organizational culture that make changing them so threatening. The challenge facing leaders of integrated healthcare delivery networks is to sensitively change these philosophical elements in a meaningful way that promises to minimize the creation of anxiety about the local organization and the network as a whole.

The chapter has also indicated that accomplishing cultural change requires both the head and heart of healthcare and physician executives. Also to be noted is that matters of the heart are not often provided by external change agents such as consultants who downsize and reengineer organizations as an analytical exercise. Executives of integrated networks must maintain a caring attitude when dealing with change. They must understand organizational culture, themselves, and others in order to be respected leaders of cultural change.

Endnote

1. The idea that there are important philosophical bases for organizational life is elaborated by Edgar H. Schein, *Organizational Culture and Leadership* (San Francisco: Jossy-Bass, 1985).

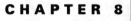

CHAPTER 8

HOSPITAL AND MEDICAL GROUP CULTURE

Network organizational dynamics that contain psychologically defensive elements can become dysfunctional when an organization is placed under stress. Network dynamics and culture have many of their origins in how healthcare leaders, executives, and employees see themselves, their organization, and their work, perceptions that can be distorted by the need to defend against anxiety. Leading the fusion of the cultural and organizational dynamics of a number of hospitals and many medical groups and related healthcare facilities is demanding and, as has been thus far explained, requires gaining an understanding of the underlying philosophical assumptions that form the basis for existing organizational dynamics and culture. Making this effort, at the minimum, shows a healthy respect for the feelings of the networked organization's employees as well as increasing sensitivity to the meaning of the asked-for changes to everyone involved.

This chapter explains how the five philosophical perspectives introduced in Chapter 7 improve understanding of hospital and medical group organizational dynamics and culture and demonstrate how to successfully change them.[1] Suggestions for change specific to hospitals and medical groups are provided to help those leading change to be more effective.

The Underlying Philosophical Assumptions of Hospital Culture and Organizational Dynamics

Traditional hospital administrative cultures introduce leadership styles, management methods, and approaches to work that are foreign and often alienating to network and physician executives and managers of nonhospital facilities. This aspect of hospital culture makes it more difficult for hospital executives and network and physician executives to understand each other. Understanding the culture of hospitals is, therefore, an important step in spanning these cultural and organization-dynamic related barriers.

The five philosophical aspects of work, as have been noted, are in part shaped by our intrapsychic processes. However, how we understand our relationship to nature, our own human nature, the nature of work, the nature of reality, and the nature of human relationships is also heavily influenced by hospital cultures. Understanding a hospital's overarching organizational culture translates into understanding its operating but not always apparent or acknowledged philosophical assumptions.

The Nature of the World of the Hospital

Understanding the world around us begins with understanding who we are. This is equally true of organizations such as hospitals. Those who lead and work for a hospital must know what the hospital is and where it begins and ends in order to understand what the rest of the world is like and in particular where competitors and threats are located. This awareness is made all the more difficult by networks that "fuzz up" organizational boundaries and make it unclear where the hospital and its contribution to the network begins and ends.

A hospital executive responsible for managing a product line such as cancer services must have a clear vision of what the hospital is including in its many parts and divisions as well as where its many parts are located in the community in order to provide one-stop shopping and seamless services to cancer patients. This understanding is made all the more difficult should the hospital become networked. A network executive responsible for network-wide cancer programs may want to incorporate the hospital's cancer service product line into the larger picture, thereby adding greater complexity, risk, and new accountabilities to the original hospital executive's mission. Care must always be taken to understand traditional boundary management issues, and the culture of the hospital and the program involved before making major changes in its design and nature.

A second aspect of the world involves beliefs and assumptions about how it works. These beliefs and assumptions can be informed and realistic, or they can suffer from some degree of personal disorganization. Leaders of a hospital who hold unrealistic beliefs about themselves, others, the hospital, and the world, can create a threatening, disorienting, dysfunctional, and ultimately nonadaptive world view, which is learned and held by many of those who work in the hospital. A hospital's leadership may consistently turn down all offers to join networks in the belief they are a passing fad and that their hospital cannot possibly lose out in the end. Their leadership may believe, for example, that being a Catholic institution will shelter them from the incursion of managed care and capitation because Catholics in the community will always want to come to "their" hospital even if there is considerable evidence that they may not be able to if the hospital is not part of the HMO they belong to. However, at the same time, managed care contracts are being lost, and the censuses is falling below 50 percent. As a result, hospital employees end up living and working in a setting that increases their anxieties rather than allaying them, which promotes reliance upon psychological defenses to block out the distressing aspects of what is going on in the world around them.

The basic assumptions the leaders of hospitals hold about the nature of the world around them are critically important and must be open to self-reflection and examination by others. If these executives feel that the world is filled with threat, as may well be the case in the 1990s, their fears will end up governing decision making and work. In contrast, the many changes occurring in the healthcare delivery marketplace today might be viewed as opportunities rather than threats and greeted with anticipation rather than fear. It is important that thoughts and feelings such as these be constantly and openly questioned to insure that they are grounded in reality as well as understood by others.

Human Nature in Hospitals

Life experience informs our beliefs about how we and others are and should be treated. A hospital executive who believes that people and groups are inherently unwilling to put in a hard day's work may also feel everyone's performance has to be monitored and evaluated as may also be the case with third-party payers. The assumptions that we hold concerning how we are and how others are returns us to an appreciation of the unconscious influence our thoughts and feelings have upon our workplace relationships. Hospital executives must be self-reflective and, therefore, aware of what they are thinking and feeling about others and the implicit accompanying basic assumptions about human nature.

Hospital executives must also be aware of the assumptions they make about the nature of their hospital and the nature of the network they may chose to join. Unrealistic and, therefore, disruptive assumptions may be held about one's hospital and the network which influence thoughts, feelings, daily actions, and decisions. A CEO may believe that his or her hospital is well run and respected in the community when that is simply not the case based upon survey data. As a result, the hospital seldom improves its services and is avoided as competitors improve their services. Care must be taken to learn about and share information, thoughts, and feelings about one's own hospital and the network in order to avoid the development of a psychologically defensive and distorted system of beliefs. Avoiding these defensive belief systems encourages reality testing, which is essential for optimum performance.

However, being grounded in reality is not always easy, and losses of grounding are not readily apparent or easily challenged by others. A CEO might be a strong advocate of total quality management principles and open participation while consistently acting to control everything and make all of the decisions. The executive does not ultimately trust others to run the hospital while, at the same time, he or she advocates a management style that is inconsistent with his or her view of others and self.

Intervening in a process such as this, while important, is also difficult. Actions such as these by a CEO may only be readily addressed by the governing board and may become unavoidable if the hospital's financial performance falters. It is also possible for a small group of executives who report to the CEO to try to tactfully raise the issue that he or she is acting in ways that are inconsistent with saying that others are trusted enough to work autonomously.

The Nature of Work in Hospitals

We all hold beliefs about our effectiveness and the effectiveness of others. We might see ourselves and our hospital as effective, powerful, and instrumental or relatively ineffective and unable to take the actions needed to survive in the marketplace. These beliefs can lead to a proactive management style or to one that is reactive and risk aversive. Management styles such as these promote feelings among employees along a continuum from feeling valued and influential to frustrated and helpless. An anxious and risk aversive CEO will tend to stifle the generation of as well as the implementation of new programs and ideas which will frustrate the most well-meaning staff members. Influences such as these become critical variables in how hospital employees understand themselves, each other, their work, and their hospital and even its role in a larger network of providers.

Hospital executives must understand their belief systems and those of their subordinates and employees in order to fully appreciate the meaning of their hospital and its work. Tight operating budgets and many operating problems may, for example, provide the basis for senior level management of a hospital to expect 70-hour work weeks from salaried managers and department heads. These employees are expected to work evenings and come in on the weekends to cover their usual workload—including that of others who have been laid off—and to answer a growing number of questions raised by the CEO aimed at tightening up operations. At the same time, information systems are so poor they make work much more difficult and time-consuming, and there are too few analytically oriented staff to support the constant requests for more research. Work, as a result, becomes overwhelming and frustrating. Many are silently angry about how they are being treated. At the same time, senior level executives are putting in long hours because they feel they have to make all the decisions. Mid-level executives and managers begin to feel discounted and cut-off from being effective as more and more decisions are made at the top. As a result, some of the better managers are leaving, and others are looking for new jobs.

Intervening in this kind of work experience begins with promoting self-reflection and inquiry on the part of senior level executives, all of whom may sense something is wrong but cannot individually do anything about it. Working for the hospital has become a negative experience. Changing this experience requires being able to discuss the nature of work in the hospital and how it is negatively affecting its employees. At the same time, the ability to work smarter appears to be blocked without the ability to upgrade information systems and decision support services. Learning to manage the stressful workloads is not the answer either. External organizational consultation may be appropriate to facilitate everyone in stepping back from the assumptions that have been made about work in order to evaluate whether they are the most adaptive ones and, if not, what assumptions are more consistent with accomplishing the hospital's work.

The Nature of Hospital Reality

Hospital executives must have accurate and timely information to be able to guide work. However, hospitals are often large and hierarchical in nature and decisions are often based on subjective data drawn from their personal experience when little information is available and when layers of filtered analyses and reports are thought to contain hidden agendas. Decision making is also often dominated by a few powerful executives at the top, which increases the threat that the subjective reality of the hospital and its staff will take over. This is especially likely during times of crisis management when there is little time to gather and test information. Also to be noted is that this type of management tends to perpetuate itself by generating more crises.

In particular, information generated by computers often seems to take on magical properties that invest it with credibility that often exceeds its true nature, which may not be particularly reflective of either the quantitative aspects of reality or, certainly, the qualitative aspects of reality. A system that, for example, measures nursing unit productivity by collecting information about a number of activities gives the appearance of being objectively collected data that can be compared to benchmarks collected from other hospitals. The result is a weekly efficiency rating that is not generated until two weeks after the end of the week. Nursing personnel, however, understand their work very differently than as reflected in the efficiency rating. The mix of variables they face, including types of patient problems, acuity levels, and quality of personnel available to them at any given time, all interact to create an experience of work that is independent of the measures being used to make decisions about resources for the nursing units. The nurses may also note that learning about efficiency problems two weeks later is of no particular benefit.

The Nature of Human Relations in Hospitals

Hospital executives and employees hold many different conceptions about how to relate to each other. In particular, the issues of autonomy and control emerge as important. Relating to powerful superiors and physicians can be threatening and infantilizing especially if they seem remote and unapproachable, which is understood to be the case if their behavior is autocratic, paternalistic, manipulative, and controlling. However, workplace relationships can also be liberating when meaningful delegation, empowerment, participation, trust, and respect exist. Hospital executives must be sensitive to those who operate the many different departments of their hospital.

A CFO of a major hospital, who is exceptionally arrogant and prone to explosive rages that publically humiliate his staff and at times others in nonfinancial areas, creates exceptional levels of animosity and tension among all of those working in finance as well as in many departments since finance affects every aspect of operations. Employees are often anxious, defensive, and irritable when it comes to dealing with finance personnel, and it is suggested the word *services* should be dropped from the departmental name Financial Services. The COO is intimidated by the CFO, and the CEO, who is also arrogant, identifies with the CFO and supports him through thick and thin.

Intervening in organizational dynamics such as this must occur from above the CEO. It is unreasonable to expect others to voluntarily subject themselves to additional abuse and possible loss of their jobs in order to do something about the situation. Rather, it is easier to either leave or knuckle under, either one of which is dysfunctional for the hospital. Members of the governing board must be in sufficient touch with the major events and processes in the hospital to learn of the problem and work with the CEO to change his or her leadership style and that of the CFO. Once again, outside consultation can be helpful in that consultants often ask the tough questions that would otherwise result in someone being fired.

The nature of the world, human nature, work, reality, and working together are the basic organizational assumptions that are hard to detect, question, and change. Their management, however, is a critical aspect of achieving excellence. Executives responsible for developing large, integrated networks of providers will have to frequently deal with the need to lead the work of organizational cultural change.

Leading Change in Hospital Culture and Organizational Dynamics

The culture of hospitals exists in ways that are not readily known or acknowledged by those who participate in them. The unseen and basically unknown nature of hospital culture, however, has a powerful influence in organizing experience and minimizing anxiety. All hospitals have a history and myths, and include unquestionable processes, ideas, and philosophies that make things more predictable and help employees feel secure but not overcontrolled.

It is, therefore, easy to understand that changing these familiar and trusted elements is threatening to employees. Change leads to anxiety as the old ways of thinking, feeling, and acting are replaced by new and unfamiliar ones. As noted in Chapter 7, hospital employees must know what the proposed change is, have time to accept it and the loss of the old way, as well as perfecting how the new way works, and they must be supported in learning new methods while adjusting to the failure of the hold way of doing work. During this transition they also have to work to master their anxieties; work through their feelings of fear, shame, and anger; and work through planning and implementing the change while, at the same time, keeping the hospital running which usually translates into working long hours under more stressful conditions. That this is a lot to ask of anyone, must be appreciated by those initiating and leading cultural change.

Hospital executives facilitate change by providing clear direction, communicating it, and pointing the way toward making the change. They must be able to understand and work through the problems and difficulties that inevitably accompany change. If hospital executives are sincere and caring, point to the way through uncertainty, provide good coaching, and celebrate successes while minimizing fault finding, they will hold their employees together while change occurs. They will help to contain their fears and anxieties by absorbing or deflecting their anger and providing a caring, nurturing, holding environment where changing is safe.

Understanding of the following leadership attributes will greatly facilitate the incorporation of change in hospital culture and organizational dynamics.

Objectivity

Objectivity is exceptionally important to maintain as those leading change plunge forward, often into a sea of conflicting feelings and distorted communication and thinking. Hospital executives must be able to identify what is important and to effectively prioritize problem solving with a certainty that reassures others. At the same time, they have to avoid the temptation of making all of the decisions, which promotes dependency.

A COO may be faced with approving one of two projects because of financial limitations. One project is from a subordinate he likes but the proposal is not well documented and appears to contribute little to the hospital's competitive advantage. The second project is from a physician who is not liked; however, the proposal is well thought through and documented and will provide competitive advantage to the hospital. A loss of objectivity in making this decision is to no one's advantage and, were it to occur, would send a clear message to those in the hospital who have innovative ideas, that unless you are on the COO's good side, your idea will not be well received.

Challenging Culture

Hospital executives must be willing to challenge the status quo because the marketplace is changing. They must be prepared to communicate clear direction and sensitively deal with resistance to change. Hospital executives must also be willing to put the hospital's interest before their own. This focus contains an element of altruism and personal sacrifice because who wants to subject themselves, their hospital, and others to change? The willingness to continually challenge the status quo has never been so much in demand as it is today. The rapidly evolving marketplace makes constant change a necessity, one that can become exhausting to lead and manage. A hard-won cancer treatment program may, after a year of operation, have to be entirely reorganized into a product line in order to be able to bid for comprehensive cancer treatment managed care contracts that require an integrated approach. Those responsible for the program may not have resolved all the operating problems with the first change, and are now faced with another disorienting change.

Inner Strength

Hospital executives must have considerable inner strength to withstand the stress that develops as employees become fearful, uncertain, angry, and resistant. Hospital executives must accept that they will become the targets of anger and aggression. They must also be prepared to persist with their change effort while remaining caring and understanding. In fact, a truly caring attitude can go a long way toward minimizing fear, anger, and aggression. A hospital executive who was responsible for consolidating several intensive care units made himself constantly available to all those involved in the change process and made every effort to make it as easy as possible. As a result, many small opportunities were spotted to improve the changes for the staff and some additional cost saving ideas were also generated. Morale remained good and those in positions that were eventually eliminated were retrained for jobs elsewhere in the hospital.

Inspiration

Hospital executives must be able to lead their employees to a new set of basic assumptions and workplace philosophies that have to be artfully developed and inspirationally presented in what becomes a constant press. Achieving this involves being able to articulate a clear idea of what the new philosophies are and how they will benefit the hospital. This is not an easy task as it requires considerable understanding of the preexisting operating assumptions and philosophies. Simply announcing a change does not work well. Of particular benefit is a statement about current philosophies as compared to the proposed new ones. This will promote reflection on what is being gained and lost by the change, which will help all concerned focus on making the needed changes. These executives must also faithfully model the new assumptions by paying attention to those aspects of organizational life that the change emphasizes. They will be carefully watched, and the appearance of double standards and inconsistencies can dependably detract from the change effort.

Participation

Hospital executives must allow for meaningful participation, which includes delegating and empowering subordinates to act to create change. They must be a good listeners and willing to work alongside those experiencing the change. Everyone must be enlisted in the change effort by the leaders.

A hospital executive who led the organization restructuring and flattening of departments also pursued the idea of empowering the remaining managers with greater decision-making authority. He thereafter steadfastly avoided making decisions that these managers were empowered to make. This behavior eventually made it clear to the managers that it was safe to make the decisions and that the executive would not feel threatened by their autonomy.

Dealing with the Symbolic

Hospital executives must be effective at dealing with the symbolic. They must be able to understand the meaning of the old basic assumptions in order to remove them and replace them with a new set of assumptions and symbols. This is particularly important when major change is planned. A typical change is to downsize the hospital while expanding ambulatory programs. While hospital employees may have the reason for downsizing clearly explained to them, they may not receive any information on why it is important to expand the ambulatory center. The results are predictable. It does not seem fair to the hospital's employees that they are the only ones who have to bear the burden of downsizing. In fact, they may come to understand that they have been bad employees, whereas the ambulatory employees must be good, as symbolized by being rewarded with growth.

In sum, this section has examined hospital organizational dynamics and culture from a number of nontraditional perspectives. Understanding how hospitals work can be seen as a function of understanding the individuals who lead them and work within them; how people who work for hospitals relate to each other; how group dynamics affect hospitals; and in the most global sense, how a series of often unacknowledged assumptions about people, nature, and work combine to create an overarching hospital culture. The understanding gained from these perspectives provides network, hospital, and physician executives with important information that facilitates working together more effectively.

The Underlying Philosophical Assumptions of Medical Group Culture and Organizational Dynamics

Medical groups also have many cultural aspects that are foreign and alienating to network and hospital executives and others who need to work with them. In particular, the prospect of shared governance of medical groups with network and hospital executives as part of an integrated system requires developing an appreciation of their organizational nature.

The Nature of the World

Members of medical groups must understand what their group is and, in particular, who its members are, how new members are added, and where its practice sites are in order to be able to separate it from the rest of its operating environment. It is easy in a large multisited group to have its members and employees focus only on the part of the group familiar to them, which causes them to lose sight of the group as a whole. Those working at a new practice site, for example, might believe they are more professional than the rest of the medical group. Although taking pride in one's work and fellow employees is natural, it is important that all members of medical groups not lose site of the larger group and its mission.

Medical groups also develop beliefs and assumptions about how work is to be accomplished. These beliefs must be grounded in reality; otherwise, the medical group risks some compromise in its performance. A typical example is confusion over whether the needs of a medical group's staff and employees take precedence over the needs and expectations of their patients. Medical group staff may not want to work in the evening and on weekends. They may make it difficult for patients to get appointments at these times, perhaps referring them to a hospital emergency room. They may also not be accessible by phone or may fail to return calls on a timely basis. Maintaining a suitable customer focus can prove difficult. When this occurs, levels of stress and anxiety usually increase for all concerned, as patients complain or stop coming to the practice.

Basic assumptions about what the medical group is and how it performs its work must be constantly examined for their validity in accomplishing the group's mission. It is also easy to lose sight of why the group exists when interpersonal and operating difficulties arise that create stress and anxiety and make working together difficult.

Human Nature in Medical Groups

Physicians and other caregivers often see human nature through a codependent lens. They often feel best about themselves when they are taking care of others. This is their calling in life, and it really is not open to inspection or reconsideration. As a result, others are often seen needing to be taken care of, and their gratitude is expected in return. This generally unconscious process is acted out on a daily basis; anyone who does not have this approach, such as hospital or network administrators, is viewed with suspicion and possibly contempt. At the same time, those receiving care are viewed as needy and dependent, and unfortunately are often depersonalized. This approach to understanding others most assuredly contains within it the seeds of considerable conflict when, for example, resources are limited or the patient's condition does not improve. It is important that physicians and caregivers be able to appreciate that their understanding of life, themselves, and others is not the only one.

Successfully working together requires finding a balance between these different points of view. CEOs of medical groups, hospitals, and networks as well as those who work with them must understand and appreciate the significance of the different views of human nature and how they can both help and hinder working together.

The Nature of Work in Medical Groups

Members of medical groups have their own ideas about how to best accomplish work as well as what work patients must do to participate in their care. Physicians are often extremely busy. Their carefully planned schedules can be easily disrupted by unplanned emergencies and unanticipated problems in carrying out a course of treatment such as a surgery, all of which can make them late to see other patients. Due to the nature of their work, physicians often cope with their own anxieties by depersonalizing their patients so they can do what they have to do without having too many feelings for them. Certainly this problem underlies the expectation that physicians should not treat themselves or their family members where objectivity may be lost. In sum, the nature of the work of physicians and those who work with them is very different from the work that hospital and network executives perform. Additionally, physicians usually love practicing medicine. Anything that detracts from this experience, including paperwork and administrative time, is not looked upon with favor. Those working with them must appreciate and accept this.

The Nature of Medical Group Reality

Physicians, physician executives, and those who work in medical groups know basically one reality, healthcare delivery. Everything else is secondary. In this regard there is often a strong concurrence of what is expected, what is going on, how to do it, and what the hoped for outcome is. Alternate realities such as the need to make businesslike decisions are, if possible, ignored. This results in a narrow focus to understanding the medical group life, which creates inhibitors to working with healthcare executives. A physician executive may steadfastly pursue the development of a cancer screening clinic despite the fact that there is little demand or support for it within the group. Members of a group may develop unrealistic perceptions of what is financially possible even though they have been presented unequivocal information that they have withdrawn all the income earned in the form of salary and that there is no capital reserve for expansion.

Changing dynamics such as these, which impose an unrealistic and narrow interpretation of the nature of reality on the management of a medical group, demands patience, perseverance, a willingness to provide concrete analyses and information, and a willingness to at times make necessary decisions that do not fulfill the preferred alternate reality. Hospital and network executives must appreciate and accept this eventuality.

The Nature of Human Relations in Medical Groups

Physicians and caregivers usually view their patients as needing to be taken care of and as perhaps inferior to them; and they relate to other executives, including their own, as potentially threatening their autonomy and mission in life. These views of others make physician executives and their colleagues difficult to deal with. A group of physicians may steadfastly feel that the management of a nearby hospital that has proposed a buyout will not honor the contract and will end up telling the physicians when and how to practice medicine. Disclaimers to the contrary are to no avail. At the same time, the physicians constantly act as though they do not need the hospital's support and can continue to practice medicine as they have in the past, despite growing financial and competitive problems.

Intervening in dynamics such as these requires persistence in explaining the nature of other realities and locating areas where they differ and where they coexist with that of physicians. It is also important for the leadership of medical groups to promote the notion of being self-reflective by encouraging everyone involved in a negotiation or the resolution of an ongoing management problem within a medical group to keep their eyes open for conflicting interpretations of reality. What is ultimately important to appreciate is that reality contains many subjective elements, not the least of which is what it means. Working together translates into developing a negotiated reality that all stakeholders and employees accept.

Leading Change in Medical Group Culture and Organizational Dynamics

The culture of medical groups exists in ways that are not readily known to or acknowledged by those who participate in them or have to relate to them. The lack of substance often makes the influence much greater than might be at first appreciated and certainly hard to identify, speak of, and change. It is also easy to appreciate that since the culture and its many elements are familiar and in fact created by its members, changing it is readily identified as threatening and distressing. Members of medical groups and their employees must understand what the change is and be permitted time to make the change, perfect any new skills that are needed and cope with their feelings about the change. They must work through many feelings of fear, shame, anger, and victimization, and they must also be able to plan and implement the changes being requested. All of these tasks when taken together are demanding for even the best of employees. Those leading the change must provide clear direction and hold steadfastly to the prescribed course of action even if there is resistance. Care must be taken to minimize blaming and scape-goating rituals, which are distracting and drain attention. Rather, the focus should be on no-fault change. Once again, the leadership attributes first mentioned in Chapter 7 are informative in the context of changing medical group culture.

Objectivity

Objectivity is exceedingly important in medical groups because of their deeply ingrained tendency to develop a monorealtiy associated only with the delivery of care. These powerful tendencies to narrow attention and conflicting information in favor of maintaining an alternate reality require the physician executives who manage medical groups to be especially cautious that they do not collude in maintaining an unrealistic view of reality, work, and others. For example, it is easy for physicians to feel overburdened with paperwork and regulation, and with the monitoring of their performance by hospitals and managed care organizations. But, rather than accepting this eventuality, they likely will develop a group attitude of avoiding and subverting these bureaucratic nightmares, which may eventually lead to their exclusion from new managed care contracts because they are not viewed as good "team" players.

Challenging Culture

Physician executives must be willing to do the relatively unpopular thing of challenging how their colleagues have traditionally seen the world, the marketplace, and the practice of medicine. Clearly the majority of physicians today have a growing disillusionment about the practice of medicine and their autonomy in treating patients. They are finding themselves limited on all sides. Hearing this from their leaders adds to the distress. However, change is no longer optional. Physician executives must be prepared to take the heat by presenting carefully developed but nonetheless distressing information and advocating change in a direction their colleagues do not want.

The best example is managed care contracting which must be done to survive, but which brings with it many practice restrictions, more paperwork, performance monitoring, and financial risks. A second example involves the growing tendency of medical groups to merge or be bought out by hospitals. Once again, this may be important for survival but these eventualities often translate into major changes for the physicians involved, starting with the loss of control over their practice.

Inner Strength

Physician executives, like their colleagues in hospitals and networks, must be willing to withstand great stress and anxiety about their decision-making skills in order to lead their medical group in change. They must accept that they will inevitably become the focus of some anger and animosity as they lead the members of their group in new and nontraditional directions. So much change must often occur that it is easy to find one or more aspects of the change process that will offend or threaten just about everyone in the medical group. The only way to succeed is through patient perseverance. Leading the development of a medical group and its participation in managed care contracting and regional networks will threaten most members of the group. Care must be taken not to further aggravate member anxieties by becoming combative and defensive when encountering resistance to the changes. Remaining reflective during these trying times will demand the utmost of inner strength and self-confidence from physician executives.

Inspiration

Physician executives must be able to lead their colleagues and employees in developing a new set of assumptions about the practice of medicine, the business of the medical group, and the harsh realities of the marketplace and politics. To do so requires a clear vision of what must be done. The vision must include acceptance of greater accountability, loss of practice autonomy, the need to constantly improve the use of clinical resources, and constant attention to meeting the perceived needs of patients. Members of the medical group must then be infused with the confidence that they can make the needed changes. At the same time, it must be clear that a caring attitude will remain and that everyone will be treated fairly and sensitively during the period of transition.

Participation

The best decision is of no value at all if no one will agree to abide by it. Allowing participation on the part of those who are interested must be viewed as both improving the decision-making process and promoting ownership of change which, in the long run, will facilitate implementation. To be avoided are manipulative efforts to provide token participation, where the leadership of the medical group of a consultant provides those participating in a committee or task group with all of the answers.

For example, a consultant-led change process created the development of a task group of more than 30 physicians and staff. The size of the group was unwieldy, which precluded its ability to be effective in planning and implementing change. The consultants then used the group as a forum for one-way communication. The result was an eventual loss of interest in the group's work and the proposed changes.

Dealing with the Symbolic

Physician executives must be sensitive when dealing with traditional aspects of practice, honored colleagues, and subspecialty turf, all of which symbolize respect and autonomy. Openly trying to discard them or denigrate these old and valued aspects of the medical group should be avoided. Rather, new symbolic images, people, and methods must be created, and members of the medical group must be permitted the opportunity to understand and attach to the new symbols of the group, which then permits the natural atrophy of the old symbols. This is particularly true of esteemed elderly colleagues who often founded the group and mentored many of its members. One or more of these physicians often symbolize many important aspects of group life such as parental authority and the ability to regenerate, grow, and learn. Group members will be exceptionally protective of these physicians. Therefore, extreme caution in developing substitute symbols will be required. There will need to be a transition of trust, respect, and authority to those who become the new symbols—the new leaders.

In sum, this section examined physician executives and medical groups using the nontraditional perspectives developed in this book. They add new insights and ways of thinking about and understanding physician executives, physicians, and the staff of medical groups. This understanding permits hospital and network executives to be more aware of and sensitive about their critically important colleagues, the physicians who make the healthcare system run.

Conclusion

It is critical to understand hospital and medical group organizational culture and dynamics before planning and implementing cultural change mandated by network participation. This understanding can be developed by interviewing members of the hospital or medical group about their work experience, hopes, fears, and aspirations. This may sound like a lot of work, but it can often be accomplished within several weeks and, if desired, by consultants who specialize in facilitating change and provide the needed research, synthesis, and recommendations to achieve successful change.

Endnote

1. This chapter is informed by the work of Edgar H. Schein, *Organizational Culture and Leadership,* (San Francisco: Jossey-Bass, 1985).

CHAPTER 9

MANAGING ORGANIZATIONAL CULTURE

Healthcare and physician executives, and hospitals and medical groups must be united into a seamless whole to create a competitive integrated healthcare delivery system. The inevitable outcome is that the nature of each organization and profession must be, in part, transcended to create the collaboration needed to optimize the entire system at the cost of potentially suboptimizing some of its parts. Optimizing the system will become a mandate as the marketplace moves toward capitation where the incentives are very different from fee-for-service and, in many ways, different from traditional managed care where volume is still important. Adjusting to these realities and being able to collaborate in their accomplishment, however, is not always going to be easily accomplished because of the psychological side of the work with its attendant anxiety and psychological defensiveness.

This book has focused attention on how the leadership styles and personalities of the executives involved in developing the merger of hospitals, physicians, and other healthcare services can make it more difficult to work together. It should be clear that there is considerable room for confusion and misunderstanding. The leadership and management styles of healthcare and physician executives and the nature of hospital and physician organizations are very different and contain elements that can readily polarize thoughts and feelings. Better understanding these potentially conflicting elements has been the purpose of this book. There is, however, one more contribution that the psychodynamic perspective can contribute to the development of integrated healthcare delivery systems. This involves understanding the nature of integration, whether it be the parts of the healthcare system or the parts of one's personality. Integration implies overcoming fragmentation, which is disruptive and pits one part against the others.

This chapter concludes the book by contrasting psychological integration with that of developing an integrated healthcare delivery organization. Discussed is the relationship of psychological integration on the part of network, hospital, and physician executives in successfully building an integrated system. More specifically, it may be hypothesized that losses of self-integration in leading the development of healthcare delivery systems will contribute to losses of system integration. Also discussed is the role of psychodynamically informed consultation to the development of organizational integration, which mirrors the usefulness of trained psychotherapists in helping their clients strive for improved personal integration.

The Need for Integration

The gradual development of an integrated healthcare delivery organization raises the question of when to start considering the nature of the emergent system. Initially, the network may have many informal elements and parts that are loosely affiliated. However, as time passes, developing a more collaborative approach and dealing with the issue of developing a fully integrated system gradually emerges. It is very likely at this point that it will be felt that the integrated system needs to develop its own identity that transcends its parts. The whole has, in a sense, become greater than the sum of its parts. This goal also implies that there is a willingness to collaborate in developing the larger enterprise.

Readiness to Collaborate

One of the key aspects in developing an integrated system is the gradual realization that all of its various suborganizations have become stakeholders, which provides them a sense of ownership of the larger organization. It is also crucial that those responsible for the network acknowledge the stakeholders and draw them into participating in the management of the network in a meaningful way. If the executives leading the development of the network, however, respond to their anxieties by trying to control them and by controlling everyone and everything else, those with whom they work will become anxious about how they are being treated (taken over) and perhaps respond with their own psychologically defensive thoughts, feelings, and actions.

The Psychodynamics and Organizational Integration

Psychodynamic integration implies that a whole initially existed and was fragmented as a result of hostile parenting where the child learned that in order to survive, it had to change itself. Lost in this change effort are parts of oneself (repressed or suppressed) while other parts may be transformed into incompatible and dysfunctional personality attributes. Psychotherapy promotes rediscovery and reintegration of these lost and transformed aspects of self, thereby promoting the development of a more balanced and complete personality. The healthcare industry was also at one time more integrated than it is now. Now, many parts of the system compete with each other working together to maintain the health of a community. The evolution toward fully integrated healthcare systems, in a sense, begins to restore the community focus to healthcare delivery. The problem implied in this process is to locate the parts and find out how they can be reintegrated into a whole that is balanced and has direction.

The advent of capitation introduces a further crises in system development: design and integration not unlike a developmental epoch such as adolescence for a young adult. Each implies a fundamental change that places the system or person under maximum stress. Healthcare delivery systems must, in response to capitation, further change their system and mix of healthcare delivery resources to focus proactively on maintaining the health of the community which has the ultimate effect of further reducing the need for inpatient care and the need to practice restorative medicine. Wellness and prevention will become the new mission and goals. This change, like adolescence, is fundamental to the nature of the healthcare system and can be depended on to introduce maximum stress, anxiety, and perhaps psychologically defensive, responses.

Psychologically defensive responses have been discussed throughout the book. Their many dysfunctional aspects have been explored. When leaders and executives become anxious and psychologically defensive their thoughts, feelings, and actions introduce conflict into working relationships. And, if the disturbances are severe enough and of a long-term nature, they can ultimately affect the entire organization. Their compulsive and unacknowledged pursuit of control to allay their anxieties can eventually alienate members of the entire organization who come to feel discounted and disempowered. These outcomes inevitably lead to resistance to change, even when it is acknowledged that change is necessary. Resistance arises then, not because of the prospect of change but as a response to the attitude of and methods used by leaders and executives to impose the change (as compared to enlisting the organization's members in discovering the need for change and how to plan and implement it).

Resistance to Change

The analogy to psychotherapy and human development can be extended one step further with some utility. Psychotherapy entails overcoming the client's propensity to resist dealing with painful life experiences including losses of self, that tend to unconsciously dominate thinking and feeling and by extension, behavior. Locating and analyzing the resistance is a window to new learning, better self-acceptance, and greater self-integration. Overcoming resistance to integration in developing fully integrated healthcare organizations is of equal significance.

Resistance to organizational change is a fact of life. Executives and employees are not often eager to give up hard-won and stable working relationships. They also are not eager to do the extra work the accompanying planning and implementation of change requires. However, change can be exhilarating and can seem to introduce new and exciting challenges and opportunities for personal growth and advancement. Change, therefore, contains within it conflicting motivations, which are likely to be greater for those who have been with the organization more than five years because they have had time to identify with it and to build up many familiar and valued working relationships.

However, the mere fact that change is needed (which may imply many kinds of change such as downsizing, rightsizing, reengineering, the development of product lines, or the implementation of total quality management) may be less distressing than the prospect that network, hospital, and medical group leaders will become autocratic and manipulative (for example, form groups that permit only token participation or espouse participation when none is really being allowed) when planning and implementing the change. Their rationale for this behavior is often explained by the belief that, in order to make change, it has to be forced upon the organization and its members—with no apologies. Top-down is the answer.

This rationale, however, assumes that the members of the organization will not be able to overcome their own resistance to change. However, as the top-down change moves forward, resistance often becomes a self-fulfilling prophesy as not only are employees unenthusiastic about giving up the familiar and predictable, they are insulted by and angry about the way they are being treated. This adds a strong new dimension to the resistance, which can lead to many key individuals leaving, taking early retirement, or dropping out of participation.

What is important about this discussion is that, while the employees may naturally experience some resistance to change because they are anxious about losing the familiar, they are made even more anxious and resistant by losses of self-integration on the part of executives who feel excessively uneasy about facing the need to lead the change. The executive's response to their anxieties is to defend against them by trying to control everything and disregarding or rationalizing feedback that contradicts the conception of themselves and their leadership as a proper approach to leading change. They, in a sense, end up creating their own alternate reality as they try to live through the unilaterally imposed change process that excludes them from meaningful participation and, therefore, alienates them from the organization, their work, others, and even from their own skills and self-image as competent executives, managers, and employees.

These outcomes and resistance to change are present in most healthcare organizations. However, acknowledging this leads to the inevitable question of what can be done to avoid the psychologically defensive outcomes and resistance to change. The most obvious step is that leaders and executives of networks, hospitals, and medical groups must learn to become self-reflective. They must be able to acknowledge that what they face would make anyone anxious and that being anxious is, therefore, normal. They must also be aware of their basic tendencies to become psychologically defensive and how these tendencies affect their leadership and management style. This book has focused on this aspect of organizational life. Another way to approach the problem, which should be considered complimentary, is to acquire external consultation in support of change. This is often indicated when senior level executives, while perhaps not particularly psychologically defensive themselves, do not have time to attend to all of the organizational dynamics created by the need for change. Understanding what is happening in the organization, whether it be a network, hospital, medical group, or some other type of healthcare service organization can be difficult for the leadership to acquire when they themselves are under pressure and in a very real sense in a glass bubble where everyone carefully observes their actions.

Consultation in Support of Change

The healthcare industry is faced with an endless supply of consultants who offer a broad array of services that can cost millions of dollars. At the same time, many of those who work in the industry question whether the consultants really add much value. At best, they are often seen as disposable hatchet men or women that permit executives to externalize the locus of responsibility for the pain inflicted in, for example, downsizing (or euphemistically, "rightsizing"). There is, however, a type of consultation aimed at enabling executives and employees to solve their own problems by facilitating their learning to be more understanding of each other, more trusting and open, and more willing to collaborate. The consultation process does not involve traditional training techniques such as team building. Rather, it focuses on all organization members learning more about themselves, each other, the group, and organizational processes.

Consultation in support of change requires the consultant be informed about the psychodynamics of the workplace in order to perform an organizational diagnosis that requires listening to organization members during confidential interviews, interpreting the interviews for signs of distress as well as dysfunctional behavior, and locating the systemic origins for the more distressing aspects of organizational experience. When the consultant believes that he or she has a clear idea of what organization members are thinking, feeling, and experiencing the next step is to design an intervention that includes discovering ways of advising, counseling, and coaching network, hospital, and physician executives and organization members to modify their behavior so as to avoid unnecessary self-defeating thoughts, feelings, and actions.

Organizational Diagnosis—
Data Collection and Interpretation

The organizational diagnosis phase includes interviews of senior management, faculty, and staff impacted by change. This phase produces a lot of information about how executives, managers, and employees are thinking and feeling about the change that is planned or already underway. In particular, the consultant learns whether those affected by the change understand the reasons for the change.

It has been said that there is never enough communication when major changes are implemented. However, there are many instances where the nature of the change and the reasons for it are poorly communicated. Relying on the chain of command is often hazardous. These hazards often prompt the use of other forms of communication such as newsletters and public forums. If employees do not understand the changes and the reason for them, it is reasonable to believe that they may not necessarily be supportive of them.

Also learned by the consultants is what individuals and groups perceive as the impact of the changes on their work lives, careers, and employment. Some individuals, groups, and departments may see little threat or direct impact of the change. The department of materials management, for example, may see little threat in the development of a new cancer treatment product line; whereas, those in the pharmacy may feel they will be faced with a major task to support the new product line. Others may feel imminently threatened such as those who work in an outdated chemotherapy infusion clinic. They may also not be sufficiently included in the change process to avoid any unnecessary damage to themselves and their department.

Those interviewed may explain why, from their point of view, it has been hard to implement the desired changes. Unbalanced attrition may be occurring, which makes it difficult to get all the work on all the shifts done. Scheduling may have become a nightmare. Lower morale may also be leading to more absenteeism, which is further aggravating the loss of staff. Unforeseeable difficulties might also be encountered, such as software that is exceptionally difficult to implement or delays in receiving new equipment.

Employees may also point out instances where there has been or seems to be a lack of insight into the interdependencies among departments, resources, and stakeholders. Major changes often result in a ripple effect that radiates out to negatively affect other departments and areas in ways not readily anticipated. Cutbacks in the numbers of nursing staff on a hospital's inpatient units may lead the remaining nurses to request additional support from other areas such as materials management to inventory floor stock and place the needed orders to replenish it.

The consultant may also learn what limitations are (real or imagined) blocking implementation. Interviewing executives, managers, and employees throughout the network, hospital, or medical group reveals much of what is happening relative to the desired change. Two types of findings result. There are those that most executives and managers recognize as business related. A list of such findings might include the observation that there was a lack of advance planning before implementing the change and that as a result many employees are uncertain about how to perform their jobs and perhaps even who to report to. Confirmation that there has been a lack of communication is common as might be the impact of unbalanced retirement of employees or attrition. These findings may only serve to confirm what the leadership knows; however, confirmation is important as are concrete examples of some of the problems. Suggestions for improvement may be made as appropriate.

The second type of findings are psychodynamically informed. They may include observations such as there has been a persistent tendency to speak of and treat one part of a hospital or medical group or one organization of a network as though it were better than another part. This is not unlike treating one child in a family as good and a second as bad. These often unconscious psychodynamics have a powerful effect: The staff of these departments or organizations eventually act them out, which splits the organization apart, making the implementation of change just that much more difficult. Some leaders, when they become anxious, as noted in this book, may resort to one or more of the psychologically defensive leadership and management styles.

Most common is to adopt a combination of perfectionistic-judgmental, arrogant-vindictive and narcissistic styles (the mastery response to anxiety), all of which can have negative effects, which are uncovered during the interviews. Grand plans may be put forward and even implemented without sufficient consideration for the need to develop detailed implementation plans. Some organization members may also report being abused and humiliated. Others may feel that the standards set cannot be met and that they are not open to further discussion or examination. Some members may believe that the only thing valued is looking and sounding good and being in control. These are all common findings that arise during an interviewing process and must be addressed by the consultant during the intervention.

Discovering Successful Intervention Strategies

The interviewing of a large number of executives, managers, and employees must be regarded as the first step in a successful intervention. The mere fact that someone has come to listen to what they have to say and provide the promise of confidentiality so that they may be frank is therapeutic in itself. Even though the consultant may do little other than ask questions, being able to vent one's thoughts and feeling is helpful, and the prospect that they will be heard by senior management adds some hope.

Organizational interventions must build upon this attitude of listening to what the employees have to say. Those responsible for leading change and those responsible for the organization, whether it is a network, hospital, or medical group, must be provided individual feedback as well as feedback as a group. Individual feedback entails synthesizing the content of the interviews and speaking of them in general terms. Questions about what any individual had to say must be refused in order to maintain confidentiality. (It is for this reason that outside consultants are more effective.) The following are typical types of feedback provided to individual executives and managers: their style is autocratic, no one appears to care about the employees, the nature of the change is not well understood, the change as it is being implemented is creating major problems, some executives and managers are not well thought of, and there may be a serious morale problem.

If the findings are sufficiently troubling, it is appropriate to also recommend a retreat by senior management to study the findings, with an eye to developing improved management of change. Retreats range from one to three days, depending on the extent of the problems. Examples of issues covered in retreats are whether the mission is clear and whether clear and measurable goals and objectives exist. Also often discussed are the nature of the organization, what type of reorganization is needed, and the nature of the planned or underway change and how best to implement it. Retreats also promote more face-to-face communication among those in attendance, which helps them bond together in a more effective work group. Multiple consultants must be available to facilitate group and interpersonal process.

The results of the individual and group interventions are made more effective by a period of ongoing consultation to individuals and groups. Individual executives may be met with to discuss their progress, and additional coaching may be provided as needed. The consultants may meet with work groups to observe their process and, when appropriate, facilitate their work. These ongoing interventions are informed by examples drawn from the diagnostic and intervention phases and build upon the agreements made during the intervention with individuals and groups as to the nature of the change needed to be more effective. Even the best of executives may tend to retreat to the use of autocratic methods (even if he or she agrees they are not appropriate) if they encounter enough stress. The consultant is there to help point this out should it occur and to help the executive or group relocate its more effective collaborative process.

Assessment and Long-Term Follow-Up

The intervention ends when the problems have been, for the most part, addressed. Individuals and groups may report that they are doing much better at collaborating, and the change may be, for the most part, implemented. At this point, it is desirable to assess the success of the many interventions. It is virtually impossible to make an accurate assessment of any one intervention because of the systemic nature of the interventions when taken together. One method of assessment is to revisit the data collected during the diagnostic phase and develop a survey instrument based upon the concerns of those interviewed. A second method is to perform a limited number of additional interviews (a sampling) or use focus groups to discuss the current experience of organization members of their life at work and to compare this information to that which was first gathered.

Long-term follow-up may also be in order if the nature of the change process being implemented takes multiple years or when the assessment shows that problems remain. The ongoing presence of a consultant permits dealing with problems that arise expeditiously (the consultant does not have to be educated by the organization again), and the consultant may observe new psychologically defensive tendencies emerging before they can produce too much organizational dysfunction (an ounce of prevention).

Conclusion

The development of horizontally and vertically integrated healthcare delivery systems is an extraordinarily difficult and demanding undertaking that will be confronted with many inhibitors, not the least of which is the psychologically defensive reactions of those involved. This book has provided a frame of reference for understanding these psychologically defensive responses and working to minimize their negative affects. This chapter has focused on an additional method for addressing these same difficulties, one which can be very effective. The use of consultants who specialize in supporting change rather than leading it or providing direction is relatively new, not only to healthcare but to all industries. Depending on the nature of and scope of the problems and planned change, internal consultants can be effective. However, when organizational distress is substantial, external consultants may be best able to deal with the many, often denied, problems that exist including those arising from the actions of top management.

In sum, addressing the psychologically defensive side or organizational life requires specially trained consultation that supports change. Although it is possible to try to meet this need internally, it is best met by locating external consultants who specialize in this work and who bring their objectivity about the organization and its dynamics to the exploration of interpersonal group and organizational dynamics as well as the ability to probe areas of organizational life that are often too dangerous (taboo) to probe from within.

APPENDIX

COMMON PSYCHOLOGICAL
DEFENSES

The following descriptions briefly explain the significance of psychological defenses and one type of personality disorder in the workplace. It should be noted that some of the defenses imply the existence of emotional energy that can be stored and released. I begin with the false self, which is a personality-like adjustment to anxiety.

False Self

Coping with feelings of powerlessness and worthlessness encourage the development of self-defeating interpersonal strategies aimed at controlling what others think, feel, and do. The child and later adult transforms self to receive caretaking and approval. A child who enthusiastically enjoys loud and boisterous play may abandon this pleasure if his or her mother becomes punitive and unavailable to the child. The child learns it is better to be as mother desires than to be his or her self.

The development of a false self undermines future development (Masterson, 1988). This split between what is actually felt and the way one feels compelled to act in order to retain love is what hurts and confuses (Bry, 1976). The child prefers to act in ways she or he believes will cause others to love and care for her or him. This self-defeating interpersonal strategy leads to distorted thinking and feeling and the impoverishing assumption of roles and behavior that promise to provide others what they want in return for being loved, cared for, and respected (Allcorn,

1991). The adult false self may, in many ways, make the perfect employee who is willing to self-adapt to receive approval.

There are many other psychological defenses that explain the intrapsychic life of an individual and his or her anger. These defenses share the avoidance of self-knowledge and recognition of the need to change, thereby assuring the need to rely upon them in the future. The compulsive and persistent nature of these reality-distorting defenses sets them apart from the norm and creates workplace paradoxes. Employees who rely upon them experience conflicting feelings and unrealistic views of themselves, others, and events. They defend the employee from painful anxiety and anger while perpetuating their use (Diamond, 1986; Masterson, 1988). These unacknowledged and usually undiscussable conflicts make psychologically defensive employees hard to work with. This is better appreciated by exploring the nature of the defenses (Coleman, 1964; Rycroft, 1973).

Denial

Denial involves being unaware of some aspects of reality or one's feelings. Past and present injuries to fragile self-esteem and disagreeable aspects of self, others, and work are not acknowledged (Tavris, 1989). The employee may calmly accept adversity that bothers others. Denial is facilitated by overworking, which directs attention away from reality and one's thoughts and feelings. Selective inattention also facilitates denial. The employee does not hear or only hears criticism. Denial is also involved in projection, which is discussed below. Denial, overwork, and selective attention all contribute to avoiding self-knowledge and the awareness that change is needed.

Emotional Insulation

Emotional insulation can lead to isolation, intellectualization, and dissociation. This defense separates feeling from thinking. An employee who should feel anger does not. Isolation separates criticism from the here and now and from oneself. No pain is felt when it occurs and perhaps never is felt. Intellectualization crowds out feelings and awareness. A threatening situation may be responded to by excessive thinking about alternatives. Finally, dissociation permits holding two conflicting attitudes or feelings. The loss of one's job may be seen as an opportunity. A dishonest executive may be an active churchgoer. An abused employee may be friendly to his or her aggressor.

Introjection

An individual may introject (take in) a good or bad self-image from others. Constant criticism and disapproval can lead to the actual incorporation of these bad self-images which then direct self-awareness. The individual may never know him- or herself to be smart enough, attractive, or skilled, regardless of evidence to the contrary. The reverse also holds true. A better sense of self can be gained by becoming like someone who is admired. Low self-esteem is compensated for by taking in the admirable attributes of others. The employee may become the ideal employee in order to be admired. Lost in this chameleon-like process is the employee's sense of true self.

Projection

Projection involves denying an unacceptable aspect of oneself and attributing it to someone else. For example, an employee who needs to feel in control may deny being controlling, instead attributing this need to a supervisor. The supervisor becomes "bad" and controlling, and the employee "good" and not controlling. Similarly, an employee who is angry about a low raise may deny his or her anger, attributing it to his or her supervisor who, it is felt, is using the low raise to get even with him or her.

Projective Identification

Projective identification involves a manager, who is the subject of the unconscious projections of one or more others, unconsciously modifying his or her thinking, feeling, and behavior to become like the projections. For example, an employee may project onto an executive those aspects of him- or herself which are powerful, knowing, and brave. This leaves the employee feeling diminished. The employee now needs to experience the executive as powerful and brave in order to feel safe. The executive is then encouraged by the employee's expectation to act powerfully and fearlessly even though this is not how her or she would normally act. If the executive accepts the expectation and begins to act powerfully and fearlessly, the executive has incorporated or identified with the projections.

Rationalization

Rationalization justifies past and present actions and disappointments. Inconsistencies and contradictions are explained away. The employee may, when treated poorly, claim that it is an accident, that everyone is treated the same way, that the supervisor is having a bad day, or, paradoxically, that he or she does not deserve better treatment. In contrast, good treatment may be taken for granted or thought to be insincere or manipulative. Discounting of this nature disposes of compliments by negating their validity.

Regression

Regression involves relying upon psychological processes, coping responses, and behavior learned as a child. An employee may begin to interpret experience in simplistic terms, have a temper tantrum, cry, sulk, and withdraw, which implies a lack of accountability. Supervisors and colleagues, it is hoped, will not take offense with the "child." Regression to an angry temper tantrum can stop or change what is happening. The employee avoids developing self-knowledge while protecting his or her self-esteem.

Repression

Repression is an extreme effort to dispose of reality. Thoughts, feelings, and events are, without awareness, excluded from consciousness. There is no awareness of the process and no recollection, although the repressed material does continue to unconsciously influence feelings and behavior (Burwick, 1981). Suppression, although similar to repression, involves an intentional effort to remove thoughts and feelings from consciousness. The content is not lost from consciousness and must be continually suppressed.

Displacement

Displacement involves discharging one's feelings (anger) in some form against objects or others who are safer from attack than the person for whom the anger is felt. A typical example is kicking a dog rather than attacking one's boss (Burwick, 1981; Madow, 1972). Another example is hitting a wall or breaking a dish.

   In sum, employees who compulsively rely upon these psychological defenses are in flight from self-knowledge and an accurate understanding of others and events to rid themselves of anxiety in favor of feeling good about themselves and, therefore, sustaining an idealized self-image and self-esteem. They are to some degree out of touch with themselves and reality. Their underlying feelings of powerlessness, worthlessness, and anger are not open to inspection or discussion. Regrettably, psychological defenses may not dispose of the experience of anxiety and may, if they are not adaptive, accentuate it.

Transference

Transference is not a defense but an additional element of the human relations that must be mentioned. Transference is a dynamic that involves the unconscious transfer of past feelings onto the present (Laiken and Schneider, 1980; Richardson, 1918). Transference creates angry disproportionate reactions to situations (Madow, 1972; Richardson, 1918). It must be noted that transference implies that anger or energy is stored and later acted upon to achieve catharsis (Berkowitz, 1962). When speaking to a female employee, a male executive may use a judgmental tone that reminds her of her father and his constant criticism. The employee may respond as she did with her father who punished her for being angry with him, by silently suffering through what the executive is saying. She feels helpless to respond and becomes anxious and defensive, reactions that have little to do with what is going on at the moment. In this example, painful and anxiety-ridden affective memory is revisited as are the associated coping responses, which are both unconsciously transferred onto the present to distort immediate experience, thinking, and feeling. In this regard, it is familiar patterns of thinking, feeling, and acting that are unwittingly reenacted as compared to stored-up energy being ventilated.

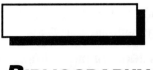

BIBLIOGRAPHY

Allcorn, Seth. "Leadership Styles: The Psychological Picture." *Personnel,* 65 (April 1988): 46–54.

Allcorn, Seth "Understanding Groups at Work," *Personnel* 66 (August 1989): 28–36.

Allcorn, Seth and Jean Allcorn "One-Minute 'Non-rewards' for Counterproductive Behavior." *Supervisory Management.* (February 1991): 10.

Astin, A. W. and R. A. Scherrei. *Maximizing Leadership Effectiveness.* San Francisco: Jossey-Bass, 1980.

Basset, G. A. *Management Styles in Transition.* New York: American Management Association, 1966.

Berkowitz, L., J. Green and J. Macaulay. "Hostility Catharsis as the Reduction of Emotional Tension." *Psychiatry,* 25 (February 1962): 221–31.

Bry, A. *How to Get Angry Without Feeling Guilty.* New York: Signet Books, 1976.

Burwick, R. *Anger: Defusing the Bomb.* Wheaton, IL: Tyndale House Publishers, 1981.

Coddington, Dean C. and Barbara J. Bendrick. *Integrated Health Care: Case Studies.* Englewood, CO: Center for Research in Ambulatory Health Care Administration, 1994.

Coddington, Dean C., Keith D. Moore, and Elizabeth A Fischer. *Reorganizing the Physician, Hospital and Health Plan Relation-*

ship. Englewood, CO: Center for Research in Ambulatory Health Care Administration, 1994.

Coile, R. "Megatrends 2000: Strategic Implications for Health Care." *Hospital Strategy Report*, 3(3) 2(July 1990): 1–8.

Coleman, J. *Abnormal Psychology and Modern Life*. Chicago: Scott, Foresman & Co, 1964.

Davies, N. and L. Felder. "Applying the Brakes to the Runaway American Health Care System: A Proposed Agenda." *Jama*, 263(January 1990): 73–76.

Diamond, M. *The Unconscious Life of Organizations: Interpreting Organizational Identity*. Westport, Connecticut: Quorum, 1993.

Diamond, M. and S. Allcorn. "Psychological Barriers to Personal Responsibility." *Organizational Dynamics*, 12(4) (Spring 1984): 66–77.

———. "Psychological Responses to Stress in Complex Organizations." *Administration and Society* (17)2 (August 1985): 217–239.

———. "Psychological Dimensions of Role Use in Bureaucratic Organizations." *Organizational Dynamics*, 14(1) (Summer 1985): 35–59.

———. "Role Formation as Defensive Activity in Bureaucratic Organizations," *Political Psychology*, (December 1986): 52–54.

———. "The Psychodynamics of Regression in Work Groups." *Human Relations*, 40(8) (August 1987): 525–543.

———. "The Freudian Factor," *Personnel Journal*, 69(3) (March 1990): 52–65.

Getzels, C. A. and E.G. Guba. "Social Behavior and the Administrative Process." *School Review*, 65 (Winter 1957): 423-41.

Horney, K. *Neurosis and Human Growth*. New York: Norton, 1950.

Jensen, A. T. "Physician Executive Leadership," *Medical Group Management*, 33(5) 33(September/October 1986): 20–30.

Knezevich, S. J. *Administration of Public Education*. New York: Harper & Row, 1969.

Laiken, D. and Schneider, A. *Listen to Me, I'm Angry*. New York: Lothrop, Lee & Shepard, 1980.

Lippitt, G. L. *Organizational Renewal*. Englewood Cliffs, New Jersey: Prentice-Hall, 1969.

Madow, L. *Anger: How to Recognize and Cope With It*. New York: Charles Scribner's Sons, 1972.

Masterson, J. *The Search for the Real Self*. New York: The Free Press, 1988.

Mazique, E. "Trends and Transformation in Health Care." *Journal of the National Medical Association*, 77(5) 77(May 1985): 365–368.

Reddin, W. J. *Managerial Effectiveness*. New York: McGraw-Hill, 1970.

Richardson, F. *The Psychology and Pedagogy of Anger*. Baltimore: Warwick & York, 1918.

Rycroft, C. *A Critical Dictionary of Psychoanalysis*. Totowa, New Jersey: Littlefield, Adams & Co, 1973.

Schein, Edgar H. *Organizational Culture and Leadership*. San Francisco: Jossey-Bass, 1985.

Tavris, C. *Anger: The Misunderstood Emotion*. New York: Touchstone, 1989.

Terry, G. R. and R. H. Hermanson. *Principles of Management*. Homewood, IL: Learning Systems Co, 1970.

Waddington, Bette A., Ed. *Integration Issues in Physician/Hospital Affiliations*. Englewood, Co: Medical Group Management Association, 1993.

INDEX

A

Anxiety, 9, 16-17, 31-2, 129, 132, 136, 159-61, 167-8, 175, 198, *see also* inside anxiety and outside anxiety
excessive, 33-4
limiting of, 118-19, 181-2
normal, 32-3
Appeals
freedom, 49-53, 60-1
love, 46-49, 60
mastery, 35-46, 60
Arrogant-vindictive versus arrogant-vindictive, 78-9, 106
intervention, 79-80, 106-7
Arrogant-vindictive versus intentionalist, 85-6
intervention, 86
Arrogant-vindictive versus narcissist, 80-1, 107-8, 112
intervention, 81-2, 108, 112-13
Arrogant-vindictive versus perfectionist, 111
intervention, 111-12
Arrogant-vindictive versus resigned, 84

intervention, 85
Arrogant-vindictive versus self-effacing, 82-3
intervention, 83-4
Autocratic group and organizational culture, 136-9
description of, 136
case example, 137
intervention strategy, 138-9
Autocratic hospital culture, 149-51
description of, 149-50
example of, 150
intervention strategy, 150-1
Autocratic medical group culture, 155-6
description of, 155
example of 155-6
intervention strategy 156

B

Basic assumptions underlying group and organization culture, 118, 159-60, 175, 186
sharing of, 119
unconscious nature of, 119

219

M

Managed care, 2

Mastery, appeal to, 35-46

Medical group culture

human nature 187

human relations, 189

nature of work, 187-8

nature of the world of, 186-7

reality, 179

see also autocratic medical group culture, homogenized medical group culture and institutionalized medical group culture

Medical group network development, inhibitors to, 22-4, see also inhibitors to collaboration

Model of psychological defenses, 32-4

N

Narcissistic leadership style, 42-5, see also case and interventions

Narcissist versus intentionalist, 90-1

intervention, 91-2

Narcissist versus narcissist, 87, 108, 113

intervention, 87-8, 109, 113-14

Narcissist versus resigned, 89-90

intervention, 90

Narcissist versus self-effacing, 88

intervention, 88-9

Nature of human relations in

hospitals, 179-81

medical groups, 189

networks, 166-7

Nature of human nature in

hospitals, 176-7

medical groups, 187

networks, 163-4

Nature of reality in

hospitals; 179

medical groups, 188-9

networks 165-6

Nature of work in

hospitals, 177-8

medical groups, 187-8

networks, 164-5

Nature of world of

the hospital, 175-6

the medical group, 186-7

the network, 162-3

Network executive function, 24-5

Network structure, 8

Normal anxiety, see anxiety

O

Objectivity in leading organizational cultural change, 168-9, 182-3, 190-1

ABOUT THE AUTHOR

Seth Allcorn, Ph.D., MBA is the Associate Dean for Fiscal Affairs at the Stritch School of Medicine, Loyola University at Chicago. He has also served as the administrator of the Department of Medicine at the School of Medicine at the University of Missouri in Columbia and University of Rochester, New York. Dr. Allcorn has published a number of books, contributed chapters and more than 50 papers on hospital administration, medical group management and the psychodynamics of organizations. Dr. Allcorn is a member of the Medical Group Management Association and the International Society for the Psychoanalytic Study of Organizations. He is a principal of Dyad, a consulting company that supports organization change.